BARGAIN BEAUTY Secrets

Tips and Tricks for
Looking Great and Feeling Fabulous

Diane Irons

author of *USA Today* bestseller *The World's Best-Kept Beauty Secrets*

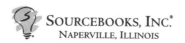

SOURCEBOOKS, INC.®
NAPERVILLE, ILLINOIS

Published by Sourcebooks, Inc.
P.O. Box 4410, Naperville, Illinois 60567-4410
(630) 961-3900
FAX: (630) 961-2168
www.sourcebooks.com

Library of Congress Cataloging-in-Publication Data

Irons, Diane.
  Bargain beauty secrets : tips and tricks for looking great and feeling fabulous / by Diane Irons.
     p. cm.
  ISBN 1-4022-0008-0
  1. Beauty, Personal. 2. Women—Health and hygiene. I. Title.
  RA778 .I7583 2002
  646.7'042—dc21

2002012082

Printed and bound in the United States of America
VHG 10 9 8 7 6 5 4 3 2 1

TABLE OF CONTENTS

DEDICATION

To the memory of my beloved grandmother, Demetria, who taught me the joys of bargain hunting and the benefits of homeopathy.

ACKNOWLEDGMENTS

I am deeply grateful for the continual support of my family, friends, and colleagues.

To all of those I have been privileged to help with their beauty and confidence, I hope that I have been helpful.

I am so appreciative of all of those who have shared their own secret bargains.

INTRODUCTION

Who doesn't love a bargain? And who among us doesn't want to look as fabulous as possible without a lot of time, money, or effort? More than any other intimate secret, we want to know the beauty secrets of other women, and we want to hear that we can afford to look the way they do.

There's an ongoing tug-of-war between wanting to look great and feeling guilty about spending a lot to do it. I have some good news for you. You don't have to spend a lot to look like you have. There are shortcuts and tricks of the trade that will get you styling without filing for bankruptcy.

With *Bargain Beauty Secrets*, you can learn how to stop making costly and embarrassing mistakes. You will expand your personal style and taste. You will begin to develop beauty radar that will get you looking better than ever while stretching your dollars twice as far.

The confidence you previously thought could only come at a high price will now be locked inside. Your looks and your esteem will soar with each decision that is certain and rational.

You'll learn the beauty jargon, the marketing ploys that push your buttons, and insider tricks of the trade that are remarkably affordable. The best news? You're going to look and feel better in the least amount of time and with little or no cost to you.

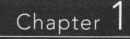

THE PRICE OF BEAUTY

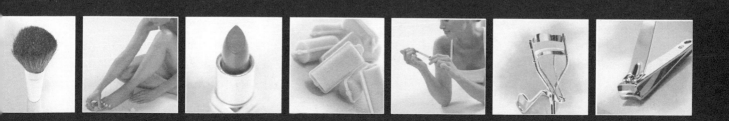

GETTING STARTED

How do you begin? You start by throwing away any previous conceptions about how beauty should look. More than anything you can put on your face or body, you need to visualize what you want to look like. You should sit down and figure out what you need to obtain your beauty goals.

TRY **BEFORE** YOU BUY

Insist on trying anything you will put on or in your body. If that's not possible, then there should be a solid customer satisfaction response.

DO YOUR HOMEWORK

Talk to friends about products that they use, the results they got, what worked, and what didn't.

FREEBIE
Don't Let Them Hook You In

You'll see pictures of beautiful models, you'll hear incredible testimonials (oh, those infomercials), and yet you need to take it all with a grain of salt. Does it sound too good? Too quick? Too bizarre? It probably is. The beauty and diet industries are multi-billion-dollar cash cows and they'll do—and say—anything to grab your attention and money.

DON'T WASTE PRODUCT

I'm not talking about measuring your shampoo or sitting on your toothpaste to get the last drop out of it. But so many of us have the philosophy,

"If a little is good, then more must be even better. Even more will really make me sizzle."

You know how they tell you to shampoo twice? You don't always need to. Trust your own beauty intuition.

THERE IS NO CORRELATION BETWEEN THE AMOUNT OF MONEY YOU SPEND TO THE VALUE OF BEAUTY BENEFITS.

GETTING A GREAT DEAL DOESN'T MEAN DEPRIVING YOURSELF

You're just learning to do everything a little differently. You can still see your favorite movie, but might consider taking in a matinee. You might not be choosing a tony day spa, but instead treating yourself to a manicure for under $10. You may not be able to invest in a new wardrobe, but be thrilled with a new scarf that feels and looks great. Going to spend big money on a beautifully scented sachet? Of course not, you can make your own in minutes.

Legendary fashion designer Coco Chanel said it best: "There are people who have money and people who are rich." You can look rich without anyone knowing your budget.

A SPACE FOR YOURSELF

Now is the time to carve out a special area that belongs only to you. Even if you are sharing a room, you should have your own bureau, or at least a few drawers. You should be keeping your things together with pride and care.

Fold your clothes and organize them by color.

Put small things like socks and underwear in shoeboxes.

Keep a box under your bed to store items like sweaters and out-of-season clothing.

Set Up New Rules of the Game

Do things **DIFFERENTLY**

EXPERIMENT with what you've got.

Become a **BLANK CANVAS**

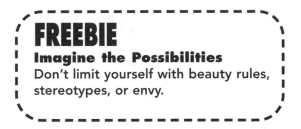

FREEBIE
Imagine the Possibilities
Don't limit yourself with beauty rules, stereotypes, or envy.

Chapter 2

CHEAP TRICKS

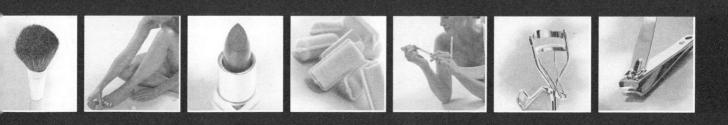

MAKEUP ARTIST TRICKS

Apply cherry lip balm in the center of your lips. Patting gloss there has plumping power (attracting the light) and it will stay longer because of its pigment.

Make a customized tinted moisturizer that matches your skin exactly. Just mix a few drops of liquid foundation or liquid to powder foundation with a few drops of instant bronzer.

Create soft definition on eyes by dabbing an eye-lining pencil in between roots of the upper lashes, and then smudging with a tiny brush.

Find the most flattering lip shade by biting your lips for thirty seconds and matching that color. Another way to choose the right shade is to match the color to the inside of your lower lip.

Pick up your blush by lightly tapping the blush with only the tips of the bristles.

Otherwise, you're not only wasting a lot of product but applying just too much. You should barely be able to see the color on the brush.

Tap your **BLUSH BRUSH** on a tissue to remove any excess.

Never stroke color across cheeks. Just smile and **PAT THE BRUSH** on your cheekbones.

To remove excess blush from cheeks, dampen a cloth and **LIGHTLY PRESS** the cloth to your face.

BARGAIN BEAUTY HEROES

Baking Soda

Use it to protect clothing from deodorant stains. Apply it after deodorant.

It's a great toothpaste. Mix it with your regular toothpaste or add it to hydrogen peroxide.

Add it to your bath to soothe irritated skin.

Vitamin E Capsules

Use them to add important moisturizing value to any inexpensive cream.

Break open a capsule and rub the oil between your hands, then pat over your hair to defrizz.

Talcum Powder

Dry shampoo your hair by dusting a small amount on your scalp and brushing through hair. It absorbs oils and adds body, too.

Eye Redness Reliever

Use it to brighten tired eyes, of course, but also rely on it to conceal pimples. Just squirt some on a cotton swab and hold the swab on the pimple for about fifteen seconds.

Hydrogen Peroxide

This is an excellent toner for acne-prone or oily skin. Pour some on a cotton ball and wipe over your face after cleansing.

Vitamin K

Break it open and use it to lighten undereye circles.

Pat it on spider veins.

Its properties boost circulation and get blood flowing.

Petroleum Jelly

Use it on eyelids to add a natural sheen.

It creates gloss from regular lipstick. Just add it on top of lipstick or liner.

Toothbrush

Use it to exfoliate your lips

Spray it with a bit of hairspray and keep your brows in place.

Brush your tongue when you brush your teeth for fresh breath.

Use it to tease small pieces of hair.

BUY IN BULK those products you know you won't stop needing. Shop on sale or at wholesale clubs for such things as deodorant, shampoo, underwear, body lotion, etc.

The **NUMBER ONE LIPSTICK** bargain is a brownish-pink color. It is the one must-have for your handbag. It works for most skin tones, and it can be used on lips, cheeks, and even eyes as a creamy shadow. Don't pick anything too dark, or it won't be as flattering.

For **SOFT HAIR**, rub in unscented body lotion. (Using anything with fragrance won't work because those products contain alcohol.)

MAX FOR YOUR CASH

Store makeup and nail polish in a cool dry area.

Keep caps on tight to prevent melting or color separation.

A **LITTLE DAB** WILL DO

All you need is a quarter size of moisturizer no matter what your skin type. Anything more is a waste of product and money.

Use your toothpaste dry. It will work more effectively and you'll need less.

USE YOUR **FINGERS**

Apply a nickel-sized dose of foundation with your fingers. Using a sponge wastes product since the sponge will absorb some of the foundation.

THE **LAST** DROP

Store remaining makeup upside down to get the last bit out. Do the same with shampoos and body treatments.

Apply nail polish thinner to an almost-empty nail polish bottle.

Dilute the last quarter of shampoos and conditioners with an equal amount of water.

Fix a **BROKEN LIPSTICK** by heating it with a hair dryer. Then reattach it and store overnight in the refrigerator.

CHEAP HAIR RINSES

A cup of chamomile tea for blondes.

A cup of cranberry juice for brunettes and redheads.

Rinse it out quickly as a final rinse with a cup of cool water. Compare it to shine shampoos that run about $8.00.

REMOVE A STAIN WITH A BIT OF TOOTHPASTE. JUST RUB IT IN BEFORE LAUNDERING.

Fragrance Ideas

There are so many ways to use fragrance, and once you start you'll want to use it everywhere, in your **BATH**, on your **BODY**, in **YOUR ROOM**, etc.

It's not necessary to spend a lot on fragrance. You can even find it in your own **KITCHEN CUPBOARD**, starting with vanilla. Put a little **VANILLA** on your hairbrush, on a lampshade, and even on your clothing.

Go to the supermarket and find great essential oils like **LAVENDER** (put it in or on your pillow to relax), and fruits like **LEMONS** and **ORANGES** to scent your bath.

Drugstore scents are lots of fun and varied. Plus, the relatively inexpensive prices allow you to **EXPERIMENT**.

Chapter 3

FOOD FOR BEAUTY

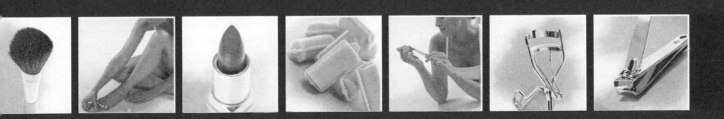

You've heard it said that if it goes in your body, you wear it. Well, here's an addendum. If it goes on your body, you can wear it, too. You'll have more radiant, firmer skin while saving a ton of money. You see, you're using the core ingredients in some of the priciest, most effective skincare products around. The difference is that you're using the product in its original form without the chemicals that need to be infused to give the product a shelf life.

AVOCADOS

Mash a ripe avocado and gently massage on undereye puffiness and dark circles. While sitting, place a cold damp washcloth over closed eyes for about fifteen minutes. Rinse off by pressing off with the cloth. The oil in the avocado is a rich moisturizer, while the cold cloth helps de-puff.

Mash a half-ripe avocado with a teaspoon of olive oil. Massage into cuticles. Leave on for fifteen minutes. Rinse.

BANANAS

Mash a banana with one egg yolk plus a teaspoon of almond extract. Apply to face and leave on until dry. Remove with cool chamomile tea to moisturize and refresh.

CHAMOMILE TEA

Use this chamomile steam treatment to clean pores and get rid of blackheads.

Steep three tea bags in boiling water for at least five minutes. Close your eyes and hold your face close to the bowl. Hold a towel over your head so the steam will go right into your face, not into the air. Follow up by cleansing in a circular motion with a coarse washcloth. Rinse and moisturize.

CHERRIES

Cherries are loaded with malic acid, which speeds up cell renewal while getting rid of dead skin cells.

Mix two tablespoons cherry juice with a tablespoon of dry oatmeal. Smooth over face for five minutes, then rinse off.

Mix a tablespoon of cherry juice concentrate with a tablespoon of sea salt. Massage over damp skin. Rinse, then moisturize. This is a great "glow" treatment for the entire body.

FREEBIE

Cornmeal has been used for generations as a cleanser and skin aid. Add water or milk to make a paste to clean and absorb grime from the skin.

CRANBERRIES

Make a cranberry cleanser. The juice is a very gentle exfoliant and acne-fighter.

Crush a handful of raw cranberries in the blender. Strain to remove pulp. Soak gauze pads in the juice and place them on your face, avoiding the eye area. Let soak in for about ten minutes, and then rinse with warm water.

EGGS

Gently take an egg white out of the shell and pat it on areas of the face that are most wrin-kled. Without moving a muscle, allow to dry on face. This works as a temporary face lift.

FREEBIE

Add an egg to your shampoo to produce volume and add shine.

GRAPEFRUIT

Grapefruit Body Scrub

Dip half a grapefruit in sugar and gently scrub over body. Shower or bathe off. Don't use this body scrub on just-shaved or sensitive areas.

The acid in the grapefruit combined with the sugar granules are very often duplicated in expensive body scrubs. It's a highly effective natural acid treatment.

Grapefruit Root Lifter

Mix the juice from one grapefruit with two cups of water in a spritzer bottle. Mist over hair while damp after shampooing. The grapefruit's acids help remove excess product buildup.

GREEN TEA

This natural anti-inflammatory reduces redness and calms irritated skin according to *The Archives of Dermatology*. Soak a cloth in cooled green tea and apply to skin for ten minutes. Then rinse away excess.

HONEY

Cleanser

Mix a tablespoon of honey with a tablespoon of finely ground almonds, and one-half teaspoon of lemon juice. Rub gently on face to cleanse.

Toner

Combine a tablespoon of honey with a teaspoon of apple juice. Smooth over face and leave on for fifteen minutes. Rinse with cool water.

Firming Mask

Mix a tablespoon of honey with an egg white. Spread over face and throat, and leave on for ten minutes. Rinse off with warm water.

Bath Moisturizer

Add one-quarter cup of honey and one-quarter cup of vinegar to your bath to smooth skin.

Smoothing Skin Conditioner

Blend together one teaspoon of honey with one teaspoon of vegetable oil and one-quarter teaspoon of lemon juice. Rub into hands, elbows, and heels. Leave on for fifteen minutes, then rinse off.

Hair Serum

Mix one-half cup of honey with two tablespoons of olive oil. Spread mixture through hair until coated. Cover hair with a shower cap and leave on twenty minutes. Shampoo out.

Acne Treatment

Mix one-half cup of warm water with one-half teaspoon of salt. Apply to blemish with a cotton ball. Maintain pressure for a couple of minutes. Dab honey on the blemish and allow to dry. Rinse off.

LEMONS

Slice a lemon in half and apply the juice to age spots.

Take the rind and put it in the foot of cut off panty hose. Tie it around your tub's faucet and let it infuse your bath with skin-softening aromatherapy.

MARGARINE

Soften skin by massaging softened margarine over your entire body. Let it penetrate your skin before showering off.

MAYONNAISE

Massage mayonnaise into hair before shampooing. Concentrate on the ends. Leave on for about ten minutes, then shampoo thoroughly. The oil and eggs in the mayonnaise make a highly concentrated and effective treatment for damaged hair.

MILK

Use milk powder and water as a paste to gently cleanse the face. The proteins in the milk make skin silky smooth. The milk's lactic acids take away dirt, debris, and the leathery layers of the skin.

MUSTARD

Create a foot bath by mixing a teaspoon of dried mustard to two quarts hot water. Soak for ten to fifteen minutes. Mustard contains stimulating qualities to relieve aching sore feet.

SOLE SURVIVOR

Warm two cups of milk in the microwave for thirty to forty seconds, and pour into a large bowl. Make sure the liquid is warm but comfortable, and soak for about fifteen minutes. While feet are still wet, use a heavy file or a coarse vegetable brush to smooth rough spots. The milk's acids will soften tough skin.

OLIVE OIL

Warm one-half cup of olive oil in the microwave for just a few seconds. Make sure it's warm, but comfortable to the touch. Massage into dry skin.

Warm two tablespoons of olive oil in the microwave until slightly warm to the touch. Apply to dry, unwashed hair. Leave on until cool. Shampoo thoroughly, and then condition as usual.

PEANUT BUTTER

Here's a food that's rich in essential fatty acids so that when applied topically can soften dry, scaly skin. Simply massage a tablespoon or two into rough patches of skin. Leave on about fifteen minutes, and then wipe off with a paper towel. Finish by rinsing in warm water.

POPPY SEEDS

Mix a teaspoon of poppy seeds with two table-spoons of jojoba oil to exfoliate rough spots on the body (knees, heels, elbows, etc.)

STRAWBERRIES

Calm irritated skin by mashing two strawberries with a teaspoon of sour cream. Apply to face and leave on ten to fifteen minutes.

Mash a strawberry, and with your finger, massage into teeth and gums—it's a natural cleaner and whitener.

SOY MILK

Researchers have found that soy milk contains an ingredient that slows hair growth. Apply it before shaving.

TOMATOES

Cut up and mash a ripe tomato. Spread it over your face and allow to set for twenty minutes. Rinse off with warm water.

Tomatoes contain lycopene, an antioxidant.

YOGURT

Soothe skin with one-half cup of plain yogurt mixed with one-half peeled cucumber and a tea-spoon of olive oil mixed together. Leave on face and neck for about fifteen minutes. Rinse with warm water. The cucumber will soothe irritated skin while the yogurt and olive oil will moisturize.

Mix one teaspoon of yogurt with one-half tea-spoon of oatmeal. Using your fingers, massage into lips, rinse, and follow up with the contents of a vitamin E capsule.

WHEAT GERM

Because it has soothing and healing properties, wheat germ makes a gentle scrub for sensitive or dry skin. Mix it with a bit of honey if you have very dry skin. Mix it with water if your skin is nor-mal. Wheat germ is high in protein and vitamins E and B.

Chapter 4

AGELESS SECRETS

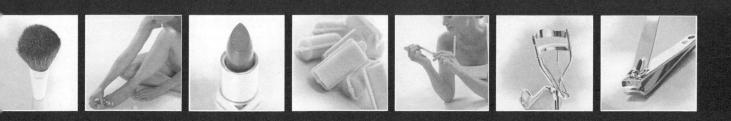

When it comes to aging, some women think that it's one or the other: the luck of the gene pool or the slice of the surgeon's knife.

There are many logical and inexpensive ways to age well and to look and feel younger than your chronological age. This chapter applies to everyone, because it's never too early or too late to turn back the clock.

There are also tips and techniques to look instantly younger and feel comfortable in your body.

In your teens and twenties, you can wear everything that's hot; you can go for all the latest, greatest trends. If your body allows, try everything that that calls your name. Just don't spend a lot while doing it.

The first place to look for trends is in discount stores.

In your thirties, you start collecting, looking for better fabrics and a more flattering fit. When you reach your forties, you start to go for well-made keepers you can live with, but you still need to add a dose or two of trend. The easiest way to accomplish this is to simply add a few trends but wear them with your classic pieces. As you reach into your fifties, sixties, and beyond, you become happy with your signature style, but you do need to update in a different way. You're still following and adding trendy looks, but in a more subdued way. You'll update with fabrics and design elements.

DON'T STAY FROZEN IN TIME

It's the number one mistake of the aging beauty. Here are some indications:

✓ It's been more than five years since you've done something (anything) different to your hair.

✓ You find that your favorite shade of makeup has been discontinued.

✓ You end up buying similar items of clothing year after year.

✓ You play it safe with the same colors, especially dark colors.

MAKING UP

Use a cream blush rather than a powder blush. It blends in much more naturally.

Rub blush upward and out along the apple of the cheeks. Stay away from the nose.

Stay away from muddy brown or gray colors. They will only make you look older.

GET YOUNGER FROM THE INSIDE OUT

You can virtually eat the years away, and what's especially nice to know is that it's much less expensive than having to buy expensive creams. There's nothing that tops beauty from the inside. When it comes to just looking good, or looking and feeling good, there's no contest.

Creams are now featuring vitamins like A, C, and E. They're used because they have the ability to fight off free radicals. Free radicals are molecules that destroy body tissue and cause wrinkling, sagging, age spots, and other exciting signs of aging. You aid the fight by eating colorful fruits and vegetables.

Brighten your smile with cranberry juice. Scientists in Israel discovered that cranberries tend to keep bacteria at bay.

FREEBIE

Mix cranberry juice with ice water if you could do without the extra calories.

The beta carotene in sweet potatoes has been known to help with vision. Bake several and keep them in the refrigerator. Microwave them and sprinkle with cinnamon when you get the urge for something sweet.

Don't forget to **DRINK THAT WATER**. According to recent studies, drinking fluoridated tap water fights osteoporosis and can improve bone density.

Be very careful about everything you put into your body. Do your very best to stay away from cigarettes and excess alcohol consumption. Smoking restricts blood flow to the top layer of the skin. This makes the skin more prone to wrinkling and sun damage.

FREEBIE

Here is a makeup artist trick to looking younger. Before applying makeup, pat a small amount of clear-drying Preparation H over wrinkled and puffy areas. It has a tightening effect that works immediately, and makes fine lines disappear for up to six hours.

STAY OUT OF THE SUN

Most of the signs of aging can be attributed to excess sun exposure.

MAINTAIN A STABLE WEIGHT

Constant yo-yo dieting plays havoc with both the skin and the body.

MAKEUP HELP

You can subtract years from your face with the right makeup. We do it all the time in the industry, but you don't need a professional with these inexpensive products.

BRONZING POWDER

Bronzing powder can go a long way in making your face look slimmer and younger. We all know how healthy we look with the glow of a suntan. But we don't want to spend the time in the sun, because in the end not only will it make us look older than those who never embraced the sun, but it puts us at risk for deadly skin cancer.

✓ Don't spend a lot. Drugstore brands are just as good.

✓ Don't try to go too dark. The shade should only be one or two shades darker than your natural skin tone.

✓ Get a subtle bronzing effect by substituting bronzer for a powder that's two shades darker than your own skin tone.

✓ Apply it where the sun would naturally color your face: nose, cheeks, chin, and forehead.

BRUSH AWAY **CROW'S FEET**

Apply pale shadow over fine lines and they'll virtually disappear when the light hits them. Try to find a shimmering foundation, or you can dip a brush into a shimmery shadow and then into your regular foundation. Literally "brush" into the lines.

FREEBIE

Give yourself an instant smile lift. Paint your smile lines with concealer, and then lightly powder over.

AGE-DEFYING RECIPES

ANTIOXIDANT **FACIAL**

Mix three tablespoons oat flour with a teaspoon of sugar and one teaspoon yogurt to form a paste. With wet fingers, gently massage mixture into skin. Allow to set for five minutes. Gently pat dry.

ANTIOXIDANT **MASK**

Cook a large carrot and mash thoroughly. Add a little milk, if necessary, to make it easy to spread. Apply to face and let set for ten minutes. Rinse.

CITRUS WRINKLE ERASER

Bring one cup milk, two teaspoons lemon juice, and one tablespoon brandy to a boil. While the mixture is warm, smooth over your face, neck, and chest area with a pastry brush. Once the mixture is dry, rinse with warm water.

This remedy helps boost collagen with its vitamin C. The brandy is known for its antiseptic powers.

NATURE'S WRINKLE CURE

Splash your face with orange juice mixed with enough water so that it won't sting (about two teaspoons orange juice to a teaspoon of water). The vitamin C helps prevent and minimize wrinkles by boosting collagen, which holds skin in place.

ANTI-AGING FREEBIES

EAT **LESS** FOOD MORE OFTEN

If you tend to skip meals, then you're more likely to gain more weight than people who eat exactly the same amount of calories distributed evenly among more frequent meals.

SLOW DOWN

It's amazing how something quite simple can make a huge difference in portion control. Try putting your fork down at least three times during the meal and taking relaxing breaths.

TURN OFF THE TV

Read a book instead. Body metabolism is at its lowest when watching TV.

CELEBRITIES SHARE ANTI-AGING SECRETS

Goldie Hawn has a special concoction she mixes up with vegetables. You can do the same by mixing your own favorite vegetables in a blender, or drink a V-8.

Rene Russo admits to keeping the years from showing with Frownies. Lots of celebrities use these sticky strips that are applied nightly to relax muscles. You also can get the same effect with adhesive tape. Criss-cross two small pieces in between your brows at night.

GET OUT OF THE CHAIR

All you need is ten minutes three times a day to do something that is more active than sitting in a chair. Window-shop the mall, climb some stairs, do something you enjoy.

START **BROWN-BAGGING** YOUR LUNCH

People who eat out tend to eat about 300 calories more than those who make their own lunch. If you tend to binge, keep toteable, nutritious food around. Put it in your refrigerator, glove compartment, purse, and even your office desk. You may include power bars, low-fat trail mix, or raisins. Make sure it's something you like.

DRESS **COMFORTABLY**

You're more likely to move if you're not constricted.

BUILD SOME **MUSCLE**

Between the ages of twenty-five and forty-five, non-exercising women lose an average ten pounds of muscle. Use free weights, vegetable cans, whatever you have around the house to build lean muscle tissue.

LOOK AT YOUR SKIN where it never gets exposed. Compare it with the areas that get constantly browned.

STAY **NATURAL**

Toxins in our diet accelerate the aging process.

CALM DOWN

Not only is it important to accept life's challenges, but you also need to accept aging.

Accept what you can't change, and instead of bemoaning what has happened in the past, discover how far you've come. Consider the stronger sense of identity you now have. Remember how insecure you were yesterday? You won't want to go back.

RELAX YOUR **STANDARDS**

You may have put on a few pounds after childbirth or menopause. If you can't get back to your high school weight, stop the battle, within limits. Never give up completely!

ACUPRESSURE FOR SKIN

This trick from Chinese medicine will help your skin to look radiant.

For seven seconds, apply pressure to the area below your jaw on both sides.

This area corresponds with the thyroid. Pressing against it releases the hormone thyroxin, which, according to Chinese medicine, keeps skin soft and revitalizes tissues. This keeps the cheeks and neck from sagging. It also helps to keep lips firm and full.

SLEEP ON YOUR **BACK**

Wrinkles can be made by sleeping the wrong way. When we sleep on one side more than the other, wrinkles can appear on that side. Avoid this problem by changing your sleep habits.

FREEBIE

Change from your regular pillowcase to a satin pillowcase. Your face will slip around the pillow, lessening wrinkling.

ANTI-AGING SUPPLEMENTS

These two supplements are at the top of researchers' lists for help with fighting wrinkles and other age-related symptoms. Check with your physician before using any supplement.

VITAMIN **C** ESTER

By bonding vitamin C with palm oil, this supplement is believed to help the vitamin go through cell membranes to target free radicals and stimulate new collagen.

DHEA

This supplement is short for dehydroepiandros-
terone, a hormone made by the adrenal glands
located just above the kidneys. Touted as "the
fountain of youth," its benefits include everything from more energy (including sexual energy) to firmer skin and thicker hair. Formerly
available only by prescription, DHEA is now sold
everywhere. It is recommended that 25 milligrams be taken starting at age thirty-five until
the age of fifty. After fifty, the dosage is recommended at 50 milligrams.

Chapter 5

WEIGHT LOSS BARGAINS

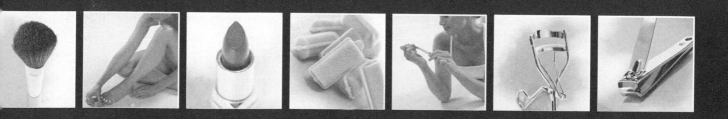

Can you lose weight without buying special foods, joining a gym, or getting involved in an expensive diet club? Yes, and you can even do it without outrageously priced supplements. By making important lifestyle changes, you'll lose the weight safely and permanently while saving money!

Get enough sleep. When you're tired, it's hard to make good decisions, especially about food.

Watch your portions. Just because you're given a certain portion doesn't mean that amount is what your body needs. Eat only until you're comfortably full. A little left on your plate each day adds up to a long-term decrease in calories.

Don't ignore your sweet tooth. A hard candy is only about 20 calories and can last up to twenty minutes. A 400-calorie ice cream cone never lasts more than ten minutes.

Personalize your program. Eat what you like, and explore new foods.

Eat during the day. If you don't, you're likely to overeat at night.

Eat breakfast. If you don't, you'll just lose energy, not calories.

LEARN TO SPICE IT UP. YOU'LL GET MORE FLAVOR FOR YOUR BITE AND MORE SATISFACTION.

Act goofy. Even if you're too busy for the gym, you can still do cardio. Put on a pair of socks, and slide around the house like a skater. You'll burn 150 calories in just ten minutes.

Don't be too hard on yourself. If you have a diet plan that's too low in calories for your weight and energy level, you'll slow down your metabolism as your body attempts to conserve calories. Don't dip below 1,200 calories or aim for more than a one- to two- pound weight loss per week.

Go for it. If you want a cookie, then have it. If you try to avoid your craving by having a slice of toast, it's not going to satisfy you.

SELF-HYPNOSIS

This is an overview of how hypnosis for weight loss works. Try it as meditation to give you similar results without the cost.

Find a place that is quiet and comfortable. Play relaxing music for two to three minutes before beginning. Picture your body exactly as you would like it to appear. See it standing before you free of all the negative eating behavior. Look at your body closely. See it as realistic but ideal. Make it a part of your own reality.

Hold that image for two more minutes. While you do, play some more relaxing music. See your body in its full size and dimensions. Now step into it. Once in, make any changes you need to feel just like you need.

You now feel comfortable in your body with no stress, and no need to overeat. Now move around in your body. Feel its strength and vitality. As you get acquainted with your new body, you get drawn into it.

Play some more music, close your eyes, and count to five. Open your eyes feeling relaxed and refreshed. This meditation should leave you feeling both positive and motivated.

SUPERMARKET SAVINGS

Stay with a list. For extra exercise, leave your cart at the end of each aisle and carry what you need back to it. This will prevent impulse purchases.

PROTEIN SHAKE

This shake is used by models and celebrities when they are dieting and needing a low-calorie/high-protein meal replacement.

1 cup raspberries

1/2 cup calcium-enriched vanilla soy milk

1/4 cup soy protein powder

1 teaspoon almond extract

1/4 cup crushed ice

Blend until smooth.

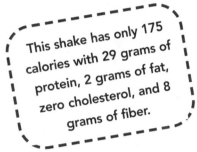

This shake has only 175 calories with 29 grams of protein, 2 grams of fat, zero cholesterol, and 8 grams of fiber.

SPA SALAD

Shhhhh…you can easily make this favorite spa recipe at home.

Sprinkle one four-ounce boneless chicken breast with salt and pepper.

Broil or grill until it's no longer pink in the center.

Cut in half diagonally.

Toss dark, leafy greens and cherry tomatoes with your favorite salsa.

Arrange on a plate and top with chicken.

Shop the produce department just before closing time. They may have markdowns.

If there's a **GREEN MARKET** around you, you might be able to get half price and better at the end of the day.

NIGHTTIME STRATEGIES

For some dieters, the evening hours bring additional challenges. Researchers have found that dark rooms and the darkness of night make us more likely to overeat.

So it stands to reason that the later you stay up, the more at risk you are for binging. The night hours are also more likely to bring about depression, which can often send us to comfort foods.

Try to schedule your bed time for an hour earlier.

If you have a favorite program that you like to watch at night, tape it. Use the nighttime hours for sleeping.

Have a meal waiting for you. You'll spend less time in the kitchen if you don't have to prepare the meal.

Take a relaxing bath.

FREEBIE
Switch to brighter light bulbs for cheerier surroundings. You'll be happier and less likely to binge.

WATER
the Ultimate Weight Loss Bargain

Reach for water before you reach for a snack. It's the cheapest, safest appetite-suppressant there is.

MUSIC THERAPY

Listen to some relaxing music when you have the urge to binge. Researchers at the Montreal Neurological Institute found that the emotional response generated by this kind of music (music that makes you feel good) activates the same feel-good center of the brain that eating your favorite foods does.

CHANGE YOUR WAYS

KEEP THE **CUPBOARDS** BARE

You'll save both money and temptation. By cutting back on the amount of food choices you have around, there will be less impulse snacking.

DO SOMETHING **INSPIRING**

A cheap incentive is sticking a picture of a dress you'd really love wear where it will motivate you. For those with a wild side, get your belly button pierced.

USE **SPICES** LIBERALLY

Ginger, cayenne, jalapeño peppers, and Tabasco sauce can boost your fat-burning ability by up to 25 percent, according to researcher at Kyoto University in Japan. According to additional studies at Laval University in Canada, the effects keep the metabolism boosted for at least three hours.

SLEEP FOR WEIGHT LOSS

Getting enough sleep does more than keep you from eating for energy. The University of Chicago recently found that a woman's metabolism rises 40 percent when she gets enough sleep.

BARGAIN SNACKS THAT ARE LESS THAN 150 CALORIES

TWO OREO COOKIES
MCDONALD'S ICE CREAM CONE
HALF CUP OF ITALIAN ICE
STARBUCKS FRAPPUCCINO ICE CREAM BAR
JELL-O WITH WHIPPED CREAM
ANGEL FOOD CAKE WITH STRAWBERRIES
FUDGSICLE

DRINK **GREEN TEA**

A study conducted by the University of Switzerland discovered that drinking green tea increases the number of calories your body burns. Try to drink three cups a day.

MORE WAYS TO CHANGE

✓ Order thin crust pizza instead of thick.

✓ Make tuna with light mayo or switch to a veggie burger .

✓ Have a Happy Meal instead of a Big Mac.

✓ Top your baked potato with salsa in place of butter and sour cream.

NEVER MISS AN EVENT just

because you're on a diet. You can go and catch up on the latest gossip, etc. You should always go for the friends, never the food.

SWITCH YOUR STRATEGY

A little of everything won't put on weight; it's those second and third helpings that will. Tell that well-meaning relative that you loved it, but you are truly full. If you don't want to eat dessert, then choose fruit. Let your good habits become the example.

KEEP A SCHEDULE

Eating at odd times can throw off your inner clock. You want to start now to set up body rhythms to work with your digestive tract. If you find this hard to do by yourself, start keeping a food journal. It will tell you when you're most hungry and need to eat.

MAKE A DIFFERENCE

Take the stairs instead of the elevator.

Speed walk on your lunch break.

CONCENTRATE

Keep food out of sight while you're:

• Watching TV

• Reading

• Studying

• Answering email

GET OUT

Try to spend twenty minutes a day sitting outside or taking a walk. If you can't, at least sit by a sunny window. Sunlight helps to control food cravings.

AT THE MALL

✓ Order a kid's meal.

✓ A yogurt is a quick pick-me-up.

✓ Have a salad without heavy dressing.

EATING OUT

CHINESE

Ask for sauce on the side.

Request foods that do not contain MSG.

Avoid buffets since the foods have more oil to keep them from drying out.

Order a stir-fried dish made with lean meat or fish instead of sweet and sour chicken or pork.

Have wonton soup instead of fried wontons.

ITALIAN

Order a side dish of pasta.

Instead of the bread, order soup. It will fill you up without the calories.

Go for the pasta with meat sauce instead of cream.

Tortellini with spinach or meat is a good choice since it requires less sauce.

MEXICAN

Corn tortillas have half the calories of flour tortillas.

Have your beans unfried.

A bean burrito has fiber to keep you full for a longer period.

Top everything with salsa. Most brands contain only 10 calories for two generous teaspoons.

BARBECUE/ROTISSERIE

Take the skin off the chicken.

Order sirloin steak or chicken with dipping sauce on the side.

DELI/SUB SHOP

Go for the roast turkey or roast beef in place of tuna or chicken salad.

FAST FOOD MENUS

You can eat anywhere as long as you make the right choices, even at fast food restaurants.

Arby's
Side salad/25 calories
Roast chicken salad/160 calories
Burger King
Broiled chicken salad/200 calories
Garden salad/25 calories without dressing
Dairy Queen
Fudge bar/50 calories
Lemon freeze/no calories
DQ sandwich/200 calories
Kentucky Fried Chicken
Mean greens/70 calories
Tender roast chicken breast without skin (4 ounce serving)/170 calories
Red beans and rice/126 calories and 4 grams of fat

McDonalds
Grilled Chicken Caesar salad/100 calories
Garden salad/100 calories
Pizza Hut
Thin & Crispy pizza with ham (1 slice)/170 calories
Subway
Veggie Delite/226 calories (without cheese)

STAY AWAY FROM cheese and mayo, and eat all you want of pickles, mustard, and ketchup.

BE CAREFUL with the toppings you choose. A perfectly healthy salad can add on calories with the wrong dressing. Steer clear of sour cream, cheese, butter, and mayo.

FREEBIE
Zero in on the vegetarian items, which usually have the least calories.

TRICKS AND TECHNIQUES

ACUPRESSURE

Stay away from the pills and other money-eating gimmicks, and try this technique to speed up your metabolism and speed digestion.

Put your hands in front of your tummy and clasp your hands, gently interlocking your fingers. With your palms touching your tummy, move your hands in clockwise circles. Repeat fifty times.

TRY SOMETHING NEW. IT WILL KEEP YOU FROM GETTING BORED.

DEVELOP NEW HABITS

Cut out your least-loved calories, and eat what you love the most before anything else. For example, if you love pretzels, enjoy them. Maybe you can live without the chips.

Don't eat in response to feelings. You can't stuff them down with food.

Don't eat unless you've made a place setting.

Give up one bad eating habit. For instance, if you eat in front of the TV or in bed, move your meal to the kitchen table.

GET MINTY FRESH

Brush your teeth and tongue with the best-tasting toothpaste you can find.

Use mouthwash and breath mints to trick your taste buds.

Always Eat
BREAKFAST

It fuels you for the day.
You'll be less hungry at lunch.

EMERGENCIES

AFTER A PIG OUT

Don't beat yourself up. It happens to everyone and it's easy to get back on track without much harm done.

Eat something

Your first thought is to skip a meal or two. This will only make you feel worse, physically and emotionally.

Get Moving

Kick up your workout to take off those added calories and for a self-esteem boost.

Take Deep Breaths

Try to clear your mind from the stresses of the day by taking deep breaths. Your stomach and diaphragm can get clenched from stress or tight clothing.

Relax with Music

It can get you in a good mood. It can make you cry. It will help you feel better about yourself by getting in touch with your feelings.

PREVENT PIG OUTS

Know the warning signs. (For example, a fight with the boss, bad news, etc.)

Have a back up plan. Make a list of things that will take your mind off food.

Make sure you reward yourself each time you win, but not with food.

Chapter 6

PERSONAL STUFF

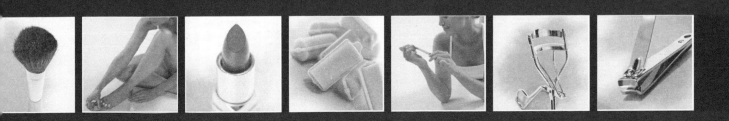

Some personal emergencies can be quickly and easily solved at home. It's good to know there are inexpensive solutions to our everyday problems. However, please consult a health practitioner if your problem worsens.

HEAT RASH

Sometimes we confuse heat rashes with acne because they can look very similar. A rash usually occurs when your sweat glands are blocked. Make sure to change clothes after exercising or spending a day outside to allow your skin to breathe.

At the first sign of the heat rash, use a medicated healing lotion.

Avoid wearing friction-causing clothing.

Keep the area that may be exposed to friction cool and dry with talcum powder.

Stay away from perfume and lotions that might react on sensitive areas.

Wear cotton clothing rather than synthetics. Cotton allows the skin to breathe.

CHAPPED LIPS

There's never a need to be a flaky kisser when you can easily make your own moisturizing lip balm.

Combine four teaspoons of almond oil and the contents of one vitamin E capsule, and warm in the microwave. When mixture is just slightly warm (check it on the inside of your wrist), gently pat on your lips. You'll love the taste!

FREEBIE

To add a bit of color to your lip balm, after the mixture has been taken out of the microwave, add a chunk or two of your favorite lipstick.

BATH BONUS

BATH ESSENTIALS

Make that soak in the tub even more beneficial by adding a few essential oils to fit your needs.

To energize: two or three drops of peppermint.

To take away stress: two or three drops of lavender mixed with a couple drops of lemon.

For PMS relief: two or three drops of geranium mixed with half a cup of very strong chamomile tea.

To boost circulation: add a cup of cranberry juice to your bath.

ADD TO IT

Rejuvenate dull, tired skin with an orange juice bath. Simply squeeze the juice of three oranges and pour into very warm water. Soak for fifteen to twenty minutes.

When your skin feels tight and uncomfortable, soften your body all over by adding a half cup of apple cider vinegar to your bath water. Soak for about twenty minutes.

Pour a packet of powdered milk into your bath and pretend you're Cleopatra. She was legendary for her amazingly soft skin, and she took milk baths every night.

FREEBIE

To ensure that you have a ring-free tub, pour a capful of baby shampoo into your bath. As the water runs, the shampoo prevents a ring around the tub. This also provides a cheap bubble bath!

TINY WHITE **BUMPS**

Get rid of those white bumps on your arms. They are clogged pores, and here's how to make them go away.

Blend two tablespoons of sugar with one teaspoon fresh lemon juice and two to three drops of vegetable oil. Rub the mixture over dry skin. The citric acid will unclog pores while the sugar whisks the debris away. The oil will add moisture. Finish by dabbing off with a warm wet towel.

BACK **BREAKOUTS**

While showering, wet a washcloth with benzoyl peroxide and wash your back.

Smooth on an anti-fungal cream.

Shrink your arms with seaweed

Go **SLEEVELESS** with pride with this easy and no-weights-required arm-toner.

Wrap sheets of **DRIED SEAWEED**, which you can find in health food stores and natural supermarkets, dipped in **WARM COFFEE** around your upper arms. Cover the seaweed with plastic wrap. Leave on for about **FIVE MINUTES** just before going out. **WIPE AWAY** with a damp washcloth.

The **SEAWEED SMOOTHES THE SKIN** while the caffeine in the coffee helps firm up arms. If the coffee aroma lingers, apply a scented moisturizing lotion.

SWEETEN **YOUR BREATH**

Here's a really effective mouthwash: steep a couple of cloves with a cinnamon stick in a small amount of water. This also can be microwaved. Let cool, and then gargle for a refreshing and natural mouthwash.

Chew a few fennel seeds. Fennel is rich in an antiseptic that destroys bacteria.

Brush the roof of your mouth and the back of your tongue every day while brushing your teeth.

Sip water often. When your mouth is dry, sulfur-containing gases normally dissolved in saliva are released into the air and onto another person.

VAGINAL **ITCH**

Avoid vaginal itch by using unscented toilet paper.

Don't overdo bubble baths.

Check your laundry detergent. It might be causing the problem.

Of course, if you do have a vaginal itch or discharge (especially with a strong odor), you should immediately contact your doctor.

ROUGH ELBOWS & KNEES

Treat rough knees and elbows to this soothing scrub. It will slough off dead skin cells to reveal new skin.

Combine three tablespoons of almond oil and two tablespoons of yogurt, sea salt, and cornmeal. Rub over elbows and knees with a vegetable brush or coarse washcloth while showering. Rinse and pat skin dry with a towel.

CLOGGED **PORES**

Use this pore-opening facial steam once a week.

Pour a cup of boiling water onto some rose petals and hold your face approximately six inches above the bowl. Cover your head with a towel so the steam does not escape. Breathe deeply for a few minutes. Pat face dry.

Calming Skin Mask

Mix three tablespoons of honey and one tablespoon of plain yogurt with enough powdered milk to make a paste.

Apply to face for fifteen minutes and rinse with warm water.

CELLULITE

Combat cellulite by mixing a cup of corn oil with half a cup of grapefruit juice and two teaspoons of dried thyme. Massage into dimpled areas like thighs and buttocks, and cover with plastic wrap for five to ten minutes. Rinse off.

STRETCH MARKS

Reduce stretch marks by rubbing them with orange rinds, and then with a vegetable brush. The bonus of using the vegetable brush is that it promotes better circulation for health and healing the system.

TIRED EYES

While you're bathing, exercise your eyes to lessen eye fatigue. Blink both sides as fast as you can fifteen times. Wink one eye at a time, keeping the other eye open. Repeat ten times with each eye.

Rejuvenate your eyes by combining a small raw potato grated with the contents of a used chamomile tea bag. Apply the mixture to closed eyes for about twenty minutes. Cover with a washcloth while you're in the bath and relax.

WRINKLES

Place your first two fingers of your left hand on the outside corner of your left eye. Pull slightly to the left to tighten the skin. Using your right index finger, massage the inside corner of the eye in a circular motion. Change hands, and then repeat on the right eye.

Before heading out the door, make sure that you smoothe on some lotion. Applying lotion **BEFORE** spritzing fragrance gives the fragrance something to cling to so it will **LAST LONGER**.

Turmeric Face Pack

Mix two teaspoons of turmeric powder with two teaspoons of warm water and one teaspoon of honey. Apply to the face. Leave on twenty minutes, and then wash off with warm water.

There are many expensive apricot kernel scrubs on the market for good reason. **APRICOTS** are rich in vitamin A, which in the industry is called the beauty vitamin. This is evident when you open an apricot pit. You'll see a soft, ivory kernel inside. It's important that you use only the inside, not the tough outer shell because it's too sharp for an exfoliant and could damage skin.

Chapter 7

BARGAIN FITNESS

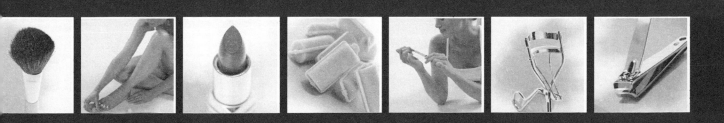

You don't have to join an expensive gym to get fit. Your main goal is to get moving!

You don't need machines to do that. Don't think of getting fit as expensive or time-consuming. Sometimes when you don't feel like a full workout, just doing a few moves can really make a big difference.

Get some free weights. It's all you need to start a strength-training regimen. Use them in the morning, evening, and during the day to keep you self-aware.

Buy a jump rope, or pull yours out of the basement. It's great exercise, and even more fun if you can remember all the rhymes you jumped to as a kid. You'll get your heart rate up and work the muscles in your upper and lower body, especially the stomach if you contract your abs while jumping.

FREEBIE

Slip the rope in your pocket and jump rope while standing at a crosslight or out in the parking lot at work during a break.

Rent or buy some exercise videos. It's like having a health club in the privacy of your own room.

Make your own ab roller by spreading out a beach towel. Lie down, and grab the ends of the towel behind your head for support.

IT'S AS EASY AS ABC

To get fit fast, models learn to cut out the ABCs. That would be alcohol, bread, and complex carbohydrates. It quickly reduces puffiness and eliminates "carb face." Do this when you need to get fit fast.

BUTT WORK

It's everyone's prime problem spot, and you can work on this problem whenever you think of it. When you're in the car or standing in line, contract your buttocks for fifteen second intervals. Tighten your muscles as you breathe in and then breathe out and release. It not only firms your butt, but relieves stress. It's the perfect antidote for heavy traffic.

KICK IT UP

Lift that butt up with a chair! Just hold onto the chair, bend one knee, and push the bottom of your foot back towards the ceiling as you squeeze. Repeat five times and then work the other leg.

SQUATS

Don't just sit in your chair; use it to tone your tush. As you lower into the chair, place your weight on your heels and contract your buttocks. Then rise out of the chair, squeezing your buttocks and tilting your pelvis forward. It's a great exercise to do while talking on the phone.

CHAIR CRUNCHING

Sit tall in your chair with your feet on the floor. Contract your abs and round your back as you lean forward. Hold for five seconds. Then sit up and repeat.

TAKE TWO

When you climb stairs, take two steps at a time. Skipping a step will force leg and buttocks muscles to extend and work harder. Plus, this movement releases endorphins that will make you feel great!

Use your **ARMS** any way you can. You'll not only tone your arms, you'll **RELIEVE STRESS** that's stored between your shoulder blades. Grab a baton if you have one.

If you've got kids, great. You can bring them to the park and **PUSH THEM ON THE SWINGS** and work your **UPPER BODY**.

HOME SWEAT HOME

Slip some specific exercises into your daily housekeeping. Do several chores at one time. For instance, make the bed, put laundry in the dryer, run upstairs to fold clean clothes and put them away.

Put some muscle into what you already do. When sweeping, concentrate to tone your arms. When you're making the beds, keep your shoulders back and pretend you have a book on your head. While you're dusting, roll up on the balls of your feet to work your calves.

Walk in place. Work your arms and put on your favorite marching music. While you're walking in place lift your knees up to waist level. Kick up your leg in front of you, working it higher and higher.

The Car Dance

While you're stuck in traffic, work your abs. Concentrate on your rib cage and pretend you're an exotic dancer. Swivel around and forget about that honker on the other side of you. Not only will you whittle your waist and harden your abs, you'll release lower back tension.

PULL WEEDS, **DIG** HOLES, **RAKE** YOUR LAWN, **SHOVEL**, AND **MOW**. **GARDENING** JUST ONE HOUR CAN BURN UP TO **500 CALORIES**.

Chapter 8

DO IT YOURSELF

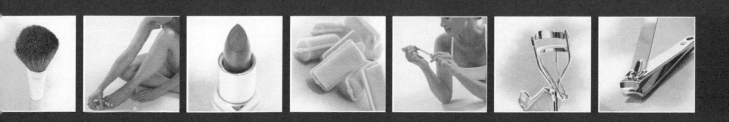

You can treat yourself at home with things you have around the house or can easily afford. It's easy to do and will empower you to take control of your looks and your life.

STEAM TREATMENTS

These benefit your skin by bringing impurities to the surface.

Fill a bowl with boiling water and lean your head over the steam. Place a towel over your head so that the steam stays trapped to go into your face, not the air.

Use a mint laxative to help clean and condition skin. Add a couple of tea bags for a toning effect. Cut up some oranges and add them to the boiling water for replenishing skin. To treat dry skin add jojoba oil (about a teaspoon).

Freshen your complexion with grape juice or red wine. Just dot it on with a cotton ball. Let it sit a minute, then rinse.

MAKE YOUR OWN BATH POWDER

Add a few drops of your favorite perfume to regular talcum powder. Shake or stir and store in a sealed container.

MAKE YOUR OWN DESIGNER BAG

Add appliqués and doilies to an inexpensive bag to create a one-of-a-kind statement of your style.

DO IT YOURSELF DANDRUFF TREATMENT

Boil four heaping tablespoons of dried thyme in two cups of water for ten minutes. Strain and allow to cool. Pour mixture over freshly washed, damp hair. Massage into scalp. Do not rinse.

Make Your Own Lip Gloss

This lip gloss is naturally sweet and will give your lips just enough color and shine. Wear it alone or over your favorite lipstick.

1 tablespoon almond oil

8 fresh cranberries

½ teaspoon honey

Mix together all ingredients and microwave until the mixture just begins to boil (about a minute).
Remove and gently mash.
Let sit for five minutes and strain through a sieve.
When cool, spoon into a clean container.
Apply to lips and refrigerate leftover gloss.

MAKE YOUR OWN
BATH SALTS

These foaming bath salts will save you a ton of money and make the perfect gift.

½ cup liquid soap

One tablespoon vegetable oil

Food coloring

6 cups rock salt crystals

2 teaspoons almond extract

Mix together soap, oil, and food color. Pour mixture over rock salt in a large bowl. Stir until crystals are evenly coated. Spread on a cookie sheet covered with waxed paper and allow to dry. Add almond extract and store in small bags.

SUNBURN **SCALP** SOOTHER

Ease the pain of a sunburned scalp with green tea. Make a cup and let it cool. Wash your hair with tepid water, and then massage the tea into your scalp. Not only will it ease your sunburn, but it gives hair a healthy shine.

MINT CONDITION TONER

Make your own facial toner by making a tea with two mint tea bags and one cup of water. Refrigerate overnight. Dip a cotton ball in the mixture and use to remove oils and surface debris.

BEFORE **TWEEZING** YOUR BROWS, DAB ON A TOPICAL TOOTHACHE ANESTHETIC LIKE ANBESOL.

MORNING/EVENING
SKIN TREATMENT

Yogurt is a natural exfoliator—it removes surface debris without taking away the skin's natural oils. Add a half teaspoon of lemon to a quarter cup of yogurt and gently rub into skin. Rinse and pat dry.

THERAPEUTIC HEATING PAD

Fill a sock with cooked basmati rice. Heat in the microwave. Apply to cramps and aches.

Use a creamy bathroom cleanser that's slightly abrasive to clean your light-colored shoes and sneakers. Just put a few drops on a cotton rag and wipe away!

MAKE YOUR OWN SOAP

These make great gifts, and making them is an easy project to do with friends.
Mix 1¾ cups of soap flakes (like Ivory Snow) with ¼ cup water.

Use food coloring to create different colors. Pour into ice cube trays or candy molds and let dry.

FABRIC MARKERS

There are lots of fun ways to use fabric markers to customize your wardrobe. Always be sure to allow at least twenty-four hours to dry before wearing.
Shirt
Take an inexpensive T-shirt, preferably new, and machine wash and dry it. Pin the edges to a piece of cardboard, flattening out wrinkles and creases. Draw a flower or a name or even your favorite slogan.
Handbag
Match the colors of an outfit to a basic bag.
Sneakers
Customize your sneakers and make a statement that's totally you.
Jeans
Add new life to an old pair of jeans with symbols and words.

FABRIC **TRICKS**

Use a glue stick to add lace to hems and pockets of a pair of cut-off jeans.

Dress up a boring T-shirt by trimming the neckline and sleeves.

Hide a stain with an inexpensive appliqué.

NO BELT? NO PROBLEM!

USE A SCARF IN CONTRASTING OR MATCHING COLORS.

TAKE A NECKLACE AND LINK IT THROUGH THE LOOPS.

RECYCLE YOUR TOOTHBRUSH AND MAKE A COOL BRACELET

Pull the bristles of your toothbrush out with tweezers. Boil the brush in a saucepan anywhere from thirty minutes to two hours until softened. Pull the toothbrush out with tongs and mold it around a bottle or glass. Stick it in the freezer and wait until it hardens. It's a great statement to put several colors on one arm.

MAKE A **BATH SACHET**

You'll need:

Knee-high nylon hose or the foot of panty hose

Fill with oatmeal, loose chamomile tea, or orange/lemon peel.

Close the top with ribbon or just knot it.

Tie it to the faucet under warm running water.

BE YOUR OWN **MAKEUP ARTIST**

You don't need dozens of lipstick shades. Instead of buying and buying, do what the most famous makeup artists do. Mix your own colors together. Not only will you get your perfect shade, but you'll also save a ton of money.

FREEBIE

Use a brush to dip into the lipstick tube. Mix colors on wax paper until you get the color you like.

GET YOUR REST

Beauty is as beauty does. Just as those partying, drug-taking models don't keep their looks, you won't either if you don't get your beauty zzzz's.

Keep regular sleep hours. Develop a routine.

Relax in a bath or shower for at least thirty minutes so you can really feel the benefits.

Start your ritual about an hour before bedtime.

DON'T WORRY ABOUT MONEY

Even if you can't afford weekly shopping binges, that's not a reason not to look fabulous. It's not important what you spend, but how you spend, and how you put things together. Some of the most fashionable models get their style by wearing vintage and thrift shop finds, and they love the thrill of the hunt.

SCENT YOUR DRAWERS
Make Your Own Sachets

Make your own sachets. You'll love the way your sweaters, lingerie, and hosiery smells when you open your drawers. Plus, these make thoughtful, inexpensive gifts.

2 pieces of fabric, about 5" x 5"

Lavender beads, rose petals, or pine needles

Needle and thread

Sew three sides of the fabric inside out. Turn the fabric right side out.

Add just enough filling so that you can still easily sew the final side.

You can sew by hand or machine.

RESPECT YOURSELF

Don't put anything in or on your body that will not benefit it in some way.

Don't deprive your body of nourishment.

Don't waste your time gossiping when you could be helping.

Be safe in who you let in your door and your life.

WHAT IF YOU WEREN'T SHY? Act for a moment like that. Take a deep breath and talk to yourself. **PICTURE** yourself speaking with **CONFIDENCE** and **GO FOR IT**.

SENSE THE **VIBES**

You know if someone is really paying you a compliment. These feelings will also serve you well in picking out an outfit or choosing your friends. Trust it.

YOU CAN'T **FOOL** YOURSELF

Trying to reason with yourself is just too easy. You've got to train your rational inner voice to win over your less rational side.

When you hear yourself saying, "I'm too busy to eat, I'll just grab a candy bar," tell yourself that the world won't stop if you pause for fifteen minutes to eat a nutritious meal.

TAKE **BABY** STEPS

When it all seems just too overwhelming, take one step at a time. When I do a makeover, I ease the client into it. As much fun as those makeovers are to watch, most of them take days but appear to take place in minutes. You need to make adjustments and tweaks as you go along. You are always a work in progress. Keep changing and you'll never be bored with your life or with yourself.

Don't take on more than you can handle!

LESS **IS** MORE

There's a big difference between subtle makeup and looking like a circus clown. Learn when to stop.

BROADEN **YOUR** PERSPECTIVE

You are not a size, a color, or a culture. They're all part of what makes you complete, but you should never be defined by them.

RECOGNIZE **ROADBLOCKS**

Don't let a remark, a pig out, or a bad hair day ruin your perspective. A slip-up is never a failure. It's an opportunity to learn what works, what doesn't work, and what needs to be done differently.

WHAT'S THE **REAL** PROBLEM?

Maybe you're eating because you're tired. Then the common sense solution is to get more rest. Are you neglecting washing your face at night because you talked on the phone too long? Set a timer so you can have time for yourself.

Don't want to miss your favorite show and you need to work out? Tape it, and feel good about yourself while watching it later.

IT'S A **TOTAL PACKAGE**

Before you waste your money on a new shade of lipstick, realize that no matter how expensive, it will only look good if you take care of your lips. That designer shirt should be hung properly and ironed to do it justice.

BE **REALISTIC**

Know that if you've never weighed 110 pounds in your life, your body is not meant to go there. Don't waste precious time trying to achieve unrealistic goals.

Find your frame size by taking your thumb and third finger and placing them around your opposite wrist. If they overlap, you have a small frame. If they just meet, you have a medium frame. If they don't touch, then you have a large frame. When you're checking out the charts, you'll see a twenty- to twenty-five-pound weight range depending on your frame.

CHECK **YOURSELF**

Knowing your body and its needs will keep you healthy and looking your very best. Here's a trick that models use to see if they need more water or moisturizer.

Pinch the skin on the back of your hand. If the skin snaps back, then your body is properly hydrated. If it stays up for a few seconds, then drink more water and apply lotion to your body. Your nails can indicate a whole crateful of problems. Splitting nails, white spots, slow growth, or thickening should be pointed out to your family doctor. Check chapter 12 and 13 on hands and feet.

ASK YOURSELF QUESTIONS

Solve your beauty dilemmas by writing down your question in the morning. Then go through your day. At night, read your question again. You will most likely have a reasonable answer. Your best answers are inside of you.

USE **ALL** YOUR SENSES

When your mind is telling you to do one thing, but your tummy is doing cartwheels, then maybe you need to reconsider your choice. Trust your gut!

AN OUNCE OF PREVENTION

It makes sense to prevent beauty and health problems as well as to solve them.

Always wash and dry your hands before touching your face.

Kill bacteria on your phone and doorknobs with rubbing alcohol or bleach.

MAKE SOME SENSE

Here are lots of "why didn't I think of that?" moments that will really make a difference:

✓Don't wear perfume when you'll be exposed to the sun. It will cause spot burning.

✓If you're going to be out all day, you'll need to reapply your sunscreen every couple of hours.

✓Don't cross your legs at the knees. It may look very lady-like, but it's putting an uneven amount of pressure on one hip and your back. Even more important, it will decrease circulation in your legs. Can anyone say "VEINS"?

✓Cover blemishes with a concealer, but make sure you seal in the concealer with a coat of powder.

✓Layer a matching shadow over your eyeliner to make the color last longer.

✓Keep your eyebrows from going all over the place by dabbing them with petroleum jelly or hairspray.

✓When wearing a bright lipstick, it's necessary to mute the rest of your face.

✓Switch to gloss at night for a dramatic effect.

✓Add sheen to your face with highlighting cream or go over your contours with a bit of baby oil.

✓Rub sunscreen over your nails to keep color from fading.

✓Use a deodorant soap after you exercise.

Chapter 9

SKIN SAVINGS

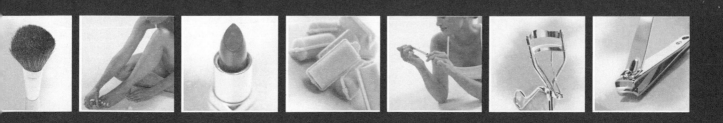

GREAT SKIN, THE ULTIMATE BEAUTY BARGAIN

Your skin is a good deal—keeping it looking great takes less money and less time than you think, and makes everything else on your face and body look better.

Not only is skin your largest organ, it's one of the most important. Your skin acts to protect the body from the environment, to allow us to feel, to regulate body temperature, and to protect organs.

Your skin is the first place to show health, neglect, and abuse. Treat it well and it will reward you with a glow and radiance that money can't buy. Just be consistent.

CLEANSERS

It's not necessary to spend a lot or to purchase an entire line of products to cleanse your skin. Quite the opposite is true. There's not even a need to cleanse your face when you first wake up. If your skin is dry, you should be able to splash your skin with water to get rid of excess oils and to reinvigorate the moisturizer you applied the evening before.

If your skin is oily, keep a small jar of powdered milk on your bathroom counter. Take a small amount in the palm of your hand, add enough water to make a paste, and give yourself an old-fashioned milk cleansing. Parisian models are legendary for their beautiful skin, and this is their secret. They would never use soap on their faces.

WATER

It's free, and it's skin hydration at its finest. The first thing you should do to get your bargain regimen started is to drink a glass of water when first awakening.

Next, splash your skin with tepid, never hot, water. Hot water robs the skin of the natural oils that have built up overnight. If you have normal to dry skin, all you need is a few splashes to remove the excess oil without stripping the skin.

If your skin is oily, you still don't need soap. The water should just be a little warmer than for normal/dry skin.

TO TONE OR NOT TO TONE?

Toning is not always necessary. And ironically, the more expensive toners contain alcohol, which may be too harsh for some skin types. The purpose of toning is to restore the pH balance to the skin and remove impurities.

Again, don't waste your money on expensive brands. There are effective and inexpensive toners that you will love.

Mixing a teaspoon of lemon juice with a half teaspoon of tepid water is my favorite toner since the lemon shrinks the pores. Also try witch hazel (available at drugstores). It's perfect for normal to dry skin and leaves the face clean and refreshed without a dry or tight feeling.

Hydrogen peroxide mixed with a little water is the toner of choice for very oily skin.

I actually prefer these toners to their cosmetic counter cousins. That they won't break the budget is just an added benefit. If you do prefer using an astringent to remove traces of dirt and for antibacterial agents, then get the most for your money by being sure that there is more alcohol than water in the product.

Stay away from toners containing fragrances, which can irritate the skin.

MOISTURIZING

Don't be fooled into thinking that a moisturizer is what gives skin moisture. Its purpose is to keep the moisture that's in your skin shielded.

CORPORATE LIES

Cosmetic and skin-care companies tell us that they've got the answer. They have that special ingredient, the secret formula that will make our skin younger, firmer, clearer, and more radiant than we've ever dreamed. And, of course, we want to believe it, so we buy the product. It doesn't work, so we go on to the next company and we buy some more. We are spending our money on yet another attempt at skin perfection. Yes, those marketers know how to push our beauty and vanity buttons so very well.

Your skin should be your first beauty priority because it's the canvas for the rest of your looks. Your makeup, no matter how expensive, can't possibly look good on neglected, abused skin. Your skin is cost-effective. Take care of it, and you'll end up spending less on corrective products like concealers, clarifiers, and the like.

The water content in moisturizers do somewhat help replenish some moisture, but it cannot penetrate the lower layers.

Don't spend a lot on a moisturizer. They're pretty much all the same. If you're looking for extra moisture, don't pay for vitamin E–added products, add your own. Take a vitamin E capsule (1,000 units), puncture it with a safety pin, and add it to a thumb-sized dollop of moisturizer. Vitamin E contains properties to help heal scar tissue and neutralize damaging free radicals. It's known as the skin vitamin. Mixing it fresh gives the product more potency.

Do the same with vitamins C and A.

Vitamin C is essential to the formation of collagen, and has been proven to protect the skin as well as fade age spots. Vitamin C also shrinks pores by helping oil-secreting glands function properly.

Vitamin A regulates skin hydration and repairs skin. It stimulates the growth of new skin cells and helps with acne.

All are available in capsules so that they can be mixed easily.

Use these added elements at night—they are not for day use. During the day, you want your moisturizer to stay on top of the skin. This keeps your makeup on top of your skin and stops it from sinking into your pores.

Give your face a treatment each time you moisturize. Tap your moisturizer into your skin. Never pull or rub. Tap up and down your face. Pressure tap under the eye area.

SKIN SINS

SUN

Use a sunscreen with an SPF of 15 to 30 and apply it at least an hour or two before being exposed to the sun. This gives the sunscreen time to interact with your skin. Remember to reapply sunscreen after swimming or perspiring. Of course, the safest tan is no tan.

SMOKING

It depletes the skin of oxygen and causes discoloration and wrinkles.

If you must smoke, at least drink a glass of water while smoking to diminish dehydration.

OVER-**SCRUBBING**

Too much of anything does not make it better. This certainly applies to what you do to your skin. Overzealous cleansing, rubbing, and scrubbing can irritate skin and cause premature wrinkling. Treat your skin like a delicate flower.

STRESS

When you're stressed out, your hormones are altered in such a way that can clog pores and cause acne.

FACIAL EXERCISES

Your face gets enough exercise with your natural expressions. If you do exercises, the muscles will stretch and then your face will drop even more.

SLEEP **STRAIN**

Not enough sleep is an enemy, and so is sleeping on your face. If you can't train yourself to sleep on your back, then by all means purchase a satin pillowcase.

CHEAP AND EFFECTIVE SKIN TREATS

CLEANSING MASK

Mix two tablespoons baking soda with just enough water to create a paste. Smooth over clean skin and leave for about ten to fifteen minutes. Rinse thoroughly with slightly warm water.

Hydrating Mask

Blend together one egg yolk, two teaspoons orange juice, one-teaspoon sour cream, and just enough oatmeal (grind it in a blender first until it becomes powder) to make a paste. Apply it to your face for ten minutes. Rinse off with warm water.

EYE **TONIC**

Use this treatment when you wake up with puffy eyes.

Cut two thin slices from a raw potato. Next, wet your eye area with saturated cotton balls. Lie down and place the potato slices over your closed eyelids. Leave them on for about ten minutes. Remove and rinse off with cool water.

FREEBIE

Always remove contact lenses and any eye makeup when using this or any other eye treatment.

SKIN **REFRESHER**

Make a pot of chamomile tea. Pour the entire pot into an ice cube tray and freeze. Pop out a cube and wrap it in a thin cloth. Rub over irritated or tired skin.

SKIN **SMOOTHER**

Mash and combine two raspberries, three blue-berries, and two strawberries with a fork. Apply pulp to clean face and leave on for fifteen minutes. Rinse.

MILK **MOISTURIZER**

Refrigerate whole milk in a spritzer bottle for about an hour. Spray over irritated or inflamed skin.

67

Skin Reviver

THIS MASK WILL WAKE UP EVEN THE MOST TIRED SKIN. SQUEEZE THE **JUICE OF AN ORANGE** WITH A TABLESPOON OF **PLAIN YOGURT**. MIX WELL AND SMOOTHE ALL OVER YOUR FACE, AVOIDING THE IMMEDIATE EYE AREA. LEAVE ON FOR **FIVE MINUTES** AND THEN RINSE OFF WITH COOL WATER.

This mask will not only deeply and gently cleanse your skin, but will leave it glowing and tingling.

FREEBIE
You can buy empty spray or spritzer bottles at drugstores and anywhere they sell artificial flowers.

FREEBIE
Save even more by mixing up powdered milk in a spritzer.

SKIN EMERGENCIES

BREAKOUTS

They can happen anywhere at any time in your life. It's big myth that if you haven't had acne as a teen you're home free.

If you've broken out in an acne rash and are running out the door, calm the redness down with a dab of aloe vera gel.

CELLULITE

Grab the strongest coffee you can find...drink it up because you need to concentrate on this trade secret emergency fix. Take the warm coffee grounds out of the coffee maker and spread it on the cellulite. Wrap up the residue in plastic wrap and roll the area over the wrap with a rolling pin. Rinse off and go!

SCARS & **STRETCH** MARKS

There are over-the-counter pads that will soften, flatten, and lighten pink and red scars and stretch marks. The success rate is quite high (about 90 percent).

Brands to watch for: Regenetrol, Curad Scar Therapy.

WHITE **BUMPS**

Usually they're located on your arms. They look like little zits, but they don't pop. They are an allergic reaction called keratosis pilaris. It usually clears up in a week, but you can speed things along.

Wash with baking soda and water. Mix two tablespoons of sugar with one teaspoon of fresh lemon juice and two to three drops of vegetable oil. Rub it over dry skin. Wipe away with a damp washcloth. The citric acid unclogs pores while the sugar whisks away debris. The oil adds moisture. Finish by dabbing the area with a warm, wet towel.

ROUGH SKIN

Mix the juice of three lemons with one cup of powdered milk, forming a paste. Rub into knees, feet, and elbows. Let set for fifteen minutes, and then scrub off with a coarse washcloth.

KNEE HELP

Treat rough knees to new skin by combining three tablespoons almond oil, two tablespoons yogurt, two tablespoons sea salt, and two tablespoons cornmeal. Rub over knees with a vegetable brush or coarse washcloth. Pat skin dry with a soft towel. Moisturize with warmed vegetable shortening.

CHAPPED LIPS

Melt one tablespoon of honey with one teaspoon of water in the microwave for about twenty seconds. Let cool and apply as a delicious lip salve.

SCALY SKIN AND RASHES

Vegetable shortening like Crisco applied to the skin will calm down rashes and deeply hydrate skin. Hospitals even use it for treating psoriasis and eczema.

Milk and yogurt applied to the skin will reduce redness.

HEATING YOUR MOISTURIZER IN THE MICROWAVE FOR ABOUT FIVE SECONDS WILL HELP IT PENETRATE THE SKIN. YOU'LL EXPERIENCE A RADIANT GLOW QUICKLY.

SKIN SAVER

If you have just a few seconds and need to look presentable, a little witch hazel followed by a tinted moisturizer will save the day.

FLAKY SKIN

Wrap some scotch tape around your finger and dab it over flakes and dry patches.

NO MAKEUP REMOVER

Use baby wipes to quickly get makeup off and refresh your face.

DROOPY SKIN

Take the white of an egg and gently pat it on clean skin. Allow to dry without moving a muscle. Blot off any excess. Apply makeup.

DEEP LINES

Mash one-half-cup papaya with one tablespoon of honey. Smooth over face, concentrating on lines. Leave on for fifteen minutes. The acids in the papaya will naturally exfoliate away the lines while the honey seals in the moisture.

ECZEMA

If you suffer from eczema, evening primrose oil may help. It contains gamma-linolenic acid

(GLA). There are skin-care products made with primrose oil, but more effective and less expensive is to purchase evening primrose oil capsules.

Break them open with a safety pin and empty the contents into the palm of your hand. Apply to eczema patches. If treating a large area, mix with an equal amount of solid vegetable shortening (like Crisco).

FREEBIE

Eat your parsley. Homeopathic practitioners claim it keeps eczema under control.

STRESSED-OUT SKIN

Take any mild salsa, purée in a blender, and apply to face, leaving on for about ten minutes. Do not use any salsa that contains peppers or spices. These ingredients can cause irritation or breakouts on the skin.

BLEMISH BARGAINS

Some of the cheapest cures can be the quickest and most effective.

Apply hemorrhoid cream to a large bump about a half hour before applying makeup.

Apply camphor oil to upper body blemishes.

Dab Milk of Magnesia on the pimple to absorb the oil and disinfect. Let it dry, then rinse off.

Take a dot of regular toothpaste (not gel) and leave it on overnight. The calcium carbonate in the toothpaste helps dry up pimples.

Hold an ice cube on the pimple for one minute. The ice constricts blood vessels that cause redness and swelling and reduces the inflammation.

Mix a teaspoon of vodka with a teaspoon of lemon juice. Dab it on blemishes with a cotton swab. It shrinks and dries out pimples and gets rid of bacteria.

Soak a piece of bread in milk. Lie down and apply to blemished area for at least fifteen minutes.

Mix a teaspoon of brewer's yeast with a tablespoon of plain yogurt and spread over pimples. Allow to dry. Brewer's yeast was used in ancient Greece for skin rejuvenation and is a natural acne fighter.

SKIN SAVVY

EXERCISE

Get a healthy glow by oxygenating the tissues of your skin with regular exercise. Don't wear a lot of makeup while you're exercising so that your skin gets a chance to clean out and "breathe."

SLEEP

Your skin rejuvenates itself in the last stages of sleep. If you're sleeping less than eight hours, you're not allowing your skin to repair itself.

A LITTLE **FAT**

You need essential fatty acids in your diet to feed your skin. Some of the models I have worked with are guilty of not having enough fat in their diet because they're afraid they'll gain weight, and it really robs their skin of its glow.

READ **LABELS**

Check expiration dates, ingredients, and follow directions for best results from your skin-care products.

HUMIDIFY

Place a humidifier in your bedroom to keep your skin hydrated while you sleep.

DRINK UP

Follow every cup of coffee and every glass of alcohol with a glass of water. The water will keep the dehydrating effects of both beverages from harming your skin.

Dull Skin Reviver

RUB A SLICE OF **ORANGE**, **GRAPEFRUIT**, **LEMON**, OR **LIME** OVER SKIN. AFTER A COUPLE OF SECONDS, RINSE WITH WARM WATER. THESE FRUITS ARE LOADED WITH **VITAMIN C AND HEALTHFUL ACIDS** THAT BREAK DOWN DEAD SKIN CELLS.

TURN YOUR **SHOWER ON HOT** AND ALLOW THE STEAM TO GO AS CLOSE TO YOUR SKIN AS POSSIBLE WITHOUT TOUCHING FOR ABOUT A MINUTE. THIS WILL CAUSE THE BLOOD TO HEAD TOWARD THE SKIN'S SURFACE TO COOL IT DOWN.

SIT ON A CHAIR AND BEND OVER WITH YOUR HANDS TOUCHING THE FLOOR. **LET YOUR HEAD GO** AS CLOSE TO THE FLOOR AS POSSIBLE AND COUNT TO THIRTY.

BREATHE DEEPLY

Stress drains your face of color and triggers other skin problems. A few deep breaths will help you unwind.

QUICK, EASY, AND CHEAP

Three of my favorite words. Put them together and you have the ability to get out the door quickly with little or no money with what you have around.

QUICKEST EVER **FACIAL**

Dip a washcloth in very warm water and apply it over your face for about thirty seconds. Quickly apply your favorite face cream to lock in the moisture.

Removing Makeup

Don't use an oily makeup remover, especially around the eye. If you have to use one with oil (for instance to remove waterproof makeup) mix it with water.

3-IN-**1** TREATMENT

In just a minute, you'll cleanse, exfoliate, and moisturize at the same time.

Combine one-quarter cup plain yogurt and one teaspoon lemon juice. Run over face in a circular motion. Rinse with cool water.

LIP FIX

Apply petroleum jelly on your lips, and gently rub with a toothbrush or washcloth.

SKIN TIGHTENER

Spread warm, wet coffee grounds on your face and let set for thirty seconds. The caffeine will tighten and firm. Rinse with warm water.

HEAL A **PAPER CUT**

Apply a drop of super glue. Then dab on petroleum jelly.

GET RID OF **CHAFING**

Apply cornstarch directly from the box to the friction points (parts that rub together). Cornstarch is an anti-chafing, extremely absorbent powder.

Get Rid of Under-Eye Bags

Wrap an ice cube in a thin washcloth and dip it in cold milk. Dab on the puffy eye area. Rinse by dipping your finger in cool water and tapping under eye again.

OVERNIGHT **SKIN** HYDRATOR

Mix the contents of a chamomile tea bag with a teaspoon of vegetable oil and a tablespoon of sesame oil. Apply the mixture to both face and neck. Tissue off any excess. Leave it on overnight. Rinse off with warm water in the morning.

ABSOLUTELY **FREE FACIALS**

Let your dishwasher give you a free facial each time you open the door and let the hot air out.

Heating water on the stove is also beneficial, but be careful!

Add a few lemons to clean out your skin. Lemons are natural astringents.

PUMPKIN SILKENER

Apply one-third cup canned or fresh pumpkin to your as an inexpensive face mask. Let it dry, and then rinse thoroughly. The natural enzymes leave your skin with a silky finish.

CRANBERRY JUICE ASTRINGENT

The acidity in this astringent will give your skin a rosy glow. All skin types except highly sensitive skin will benefit.

Combine one-quarter cup of pure cranberry juice (not juice cocktail) with one tablespoon of vodka and one tablespoon of witch hazel. Apply to skin with a cotton pad.

How to Use a Mask

Masks are a relaxing treatment that can help clean pores, absorb oils, and give the skin a radiant glow. There are dozens of masks in this and other chapters. These "do it yourself" bargain masks all require the same rules:

Wash your face. Masks work best when they're applied to clean, dry skin.

Follow directions. Don't keep a mask on longer than suggested. Keeping it on too briefly will be a waste of time and money.

Rinse your face thoroughly with warm water after removing your mask.

WHAT ARE THE BENEFITS OF PUTTING FOOD ON YOUR FACE?

If you use a homemade food mask, you get the full potency of the food including its benefits without the chemicals, the preservatives, fragrances, and other unpleasant surprises. Feel better, look great, and save a ton of money. Now that's really beautiful!

Chapter 10

MAKING UP FOR LESS

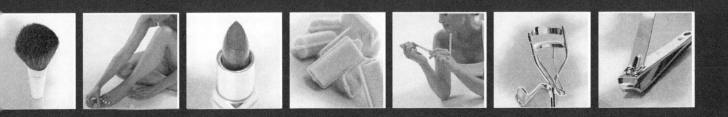

SPEND LESS, USE LESS

You don't have to spend a lot of time or money making up. The whole industry has been over-rated and under-scrutinized. First, everybody looks better with less cosmetics on their face. Second, a lot of what you're paying for is for packaging, marketing, and the space that the cosmetic companies must lease from the department stores. Oh, and did I forget those counter people?

THINK OF MAKEUP AS AN INEXPENSIVE ACCESSORY

Don't spend money on cosmetics that are trendy or bizarre.

Shop drugstores for the color of the season.

Look for high-quality, low-priced cosmetic brushes at art supply shops.

COSTLY MISTAKES

Even the very best products, used incorrectly, can become your worst enemy.

CONCEALER

Trying to fake perfect skin with concealer never works. Piling it on is like directing a sign to the imperfection that you're trying to hide.

A small dab goes a long way. More important is the color you use. Using a concealer that's too light gives off a ghostly glow. Using a concealer that's too dark makes you look like a dressed up raccoon.

LIP PENCIL

Here's a product that can look really good or just plain awful. Its purpose is to give the lips definition and keep lipstick from bleeding. Using it to outline your lips is a big no-no. It leaves a big ring around the mouth when lipstick fades. Always use a lipliner close to your lipstick shade. If you really want to save money, buy one lipliner in a neutral shade that matches your lips. In this way when lipstick eventually wears off, it will leave your lips with a slight definition and no unsightly lines.

If you are NOT COMFORTABLE with your smile, you may not feel comfortable with a very dark lipstick because it will bring too much ATTENTION to your mouth. Stay with LIPGLOSS.

BRONZER

This wonderful product is the ultimate case of too much of anything is just too much. Its purpose is to give the illusion of a healthy tan without the dangerous sun. But the problem is that it's not a tan, and it shouldn't be used as a substitute.

Use your bronzer only on the spots where the sun would hit your face naturally. That would be lightly on the cheeks, lightly on the nose and forehead, and ever so lightly on the chin.

BLUSH

So many well-intended beauties attempt to sculpt their faces with blush. It never looks right. Neither can you create high cheekbones with blush. Its sole purpose is to add color to the cheeks. That's only to the cheeks. Smile. The two rounded areas on your face are the apples, the only place that blush belongs. It should be applied after foundation and powder.

FOUNDATION

Don't wear a foundation that's too light in an attempt to even out a fading tan. Don't use a foundation that's too dark to create a tan. Get the color that literally disappears into the area right above your jaw. That's your shade.

If you really love BRIGHT COLORS, keep them to one area of your face. In this way you'll be able to wear a bright color without looking like a clown.

THE PERFECT SHADE

The biggest money drain when it comes to cosmetics is getting the wrong shade—you can't use it so you throw it away or stick it in the back of your makeup drawer.

This is probably the reason most of us don't feel comfortable shopping without a salesperson. You can become your own beauty expert. After all, who knows your face better than you?

USE YOUR **HANDS**

Actually, it's on the underside of your wrists. That's where skin undertones are most apparent.

Those with **warm** tones should go with yellow and orange shades. Those with **cool** tones should use red and blue shades.

CHECK YOUR **VEINS**

If the veins on your inner wrist are a greenish shade, then you're a warm.

Bluer veins mean you have cool tones.

THE **SCARF** TEST

Tie a pink scarf, then an orange scarf around your neck. If the orange scarf looks better, you probably look best in gold or yellow tones. If you look better in the pink scarf, pink undertones will work better for you.

This applies to everyone regardless of eye color, hair color, or ethnicity.

Fair skin usually looks best in blue-based shades.

Medium skin can wear most shades.

Dark skin is most flattered by yellow-based shades and true red lipsticks.

TRY ON SOME **JEWELRY**

Slip on a gold necklace, then a silver one.

If the gold looks better then your skin tones are warm.

Does the silver look better? You're cool.

Never a Bargain No Matter How Cheap

Dark lipliner. The obvious rim it leaves is the number one beauty blunder.

SHOPPING SAVVY

Shop where you can make returns. Keep your receipts until you're sure your new makeup is right for you. Most drugstores and cosmetic counters honor this policy.

Get samples if you can, or use the in-store testers and wear the product home to see how it looks in your own bathroom mirror or outside.

Pick two or three shades that match your skin. Draw a streak on your jawline, and see which matches best. If there's no tester, hold the bottles up to your jaw. When you can't decide between two shades, choose the slightly darker one.

FOUNDATION BASICS

Getting the right foundation is critical to the entire look. It's like building a house.

TINTED MOISTURIZER

This is the lightest foundation, with very little coverage. Smooth it over your face as you would a moisturizer.

LIQUID FOUNDATION

Gives a sheer coverage and leaves time for blending.

STICK FOUNDATION

A cream foundation with medium coverage.
It also can be used as a concealer.

CREAM TO POWDER

A non-oily foundation that dries to a matte finish. Apply it with a sponge.

FOUNDATION POWDER

A two-in-one foundation that can be used with a damp sponge for heavy coverage or with a brush for a lighter finish.

FOUNDATION APPLICATION

Become a makeup artist by combining two or even three shades of foundation to get the color you need. Always mix it in the palm of your hand, never on your face. You pay a cosmetic counter person to do this, but you'll save a bunch by mixing your own.

Start with perfectly clean skin and a little bit of moisturizer to help you spread the foundation. Dot first on blemishes or reddened areas. Begin in the middle of the face, smoothing with clean fingers or a sponge. Extend the foundation to under the chin. Apply extra foundation or concealer if needed. Only apply powder to extra oily areas, like the nose and chin.

TAN AWAY

Bronzing your skin is easier than ever. A fake tan can make you look thinner and even disguises scars and bruises. Bronzing is an excellent way to get a healthy and natural glow.

MAKE **CIRCLES**

Apply self tanner with round, circular motions.

REMOVE ANY EXCESS

Wash your hands right after applying. If any stains remain, wipe off with cuticle remover.

Brush excess over upper lip, earlobes, upper ears, and upper chest.

QUICK AND CHEAP FIXES

SMOOTH LINES

Use the product on the inside of the cap of your liquid foundation and apply directly on lines with a brush or sponge.

LIGHTEN **DARK SPOTS**

Paint concealer on with a brush after applying foundation. Keep layering until you get the desired effect. Then pat around it with your finger to blend.

ERASE **DARK** CIRCLES

If the area has a pinkish cast, add a little green eye shadow to your concealer and pat it on.

If the circle has a blue tinge, then use a pink shadow mixed with concealer or foundation.

TAKE AWAY **SHINE**

Separate a tissue into two pieces and blot oil and shine away. This will also blend back streaky foundation.

KEEP YOUR MAKE UP ON **ALL DAY**

Apply cornstarch before applying foundation. It will keep it from slipping off. Use a brush or a puff, and use the cornstarch right from the box.

MULTI USE PRODUCTS

You can save a ton of money by finding products that have more than one use. For instance, your blush can be used as a topcoat for your lipstick. In a soft neutral shade your blush is an eye-awakening shadow.

MAKING EYES

EYEBROWS

They are an important part of the total face. As a rule, they should be one or two shades darker than your hair color.

Don't go crazy with the tweezers, but you don't want to ever leave them unruly. If you're unsure about what to do, get a stencil kit, or let a professional do it for you.

If you're too nervous to tweeze, brush your brows up and snip any hairs that go above the brow with a small pair of scissors.

Always place a little gel on your brows.

SPRAY A **TOOTHBRUSH** WITH **HAIR SPRAY** TO HOLD YOUR BROWS IN PLACE.

Choose Thick Brows
- If your face is round or heart shaped
- Your nose is thick or wide
- You have large or wide-set eyes.
- You don't want a lot of maintenance

Choose Thin Brows
- If your face is long and thin
- Your eyes are close or deep-set
- Your forehead is small
- You have small features

Make your brows look even more **DRAMATIC** by running a pink or white pencil under the arch.

SHADOW TIPS

Keep your eye shadow from creasing by powdering the eyelid first. Creasing happens when the natural oils in your skin mix with the eye shadow, causing the shadow to collect in the folds of your upper lids.

LASHES

It's easy to make any lash look fuller.

With the pad of your pointer finger, gently pull on the corner of the eye just enough so that skin is smooth and taut. Add a thin line of dark powder shadow directly on top of your actual lash line. Concentrate your mascara at the base of your lashes with a back and forth motion. Then sweep the entire length of the lash once.

Black mascara gives the most drama to your eyes. For parties, you can use the same black mascara dipped into a colored shadow. For the office or weekends, you might prefer brown mascara or even clear mascara (it doubles as a brow fix). It also may be a better look for you if you're a natural blonde or light redhead.

LINING EYES

It takes practice and a steady hand to apply eyeliner. Here are the steps that will take you there.

Dust powder over lids if you don't already have eye shadow on. If you plan to curl your lashes, do it before lining eyes. Otherwise, you'll smudge the line. Choose the right formula. For a clean, straight line use a cake or liquid liner. To create a soft line, use eyeliner pencil. Rest your elbow on a hard surface to steady your hand. Start in the middle of the eyelid and draw as close to the lashes as possible. First apply the liner toward the inner corner of your eye. Then draw to the outer end of the eye with a slightly upward turn at the end.

EYE TRICKS

To "smoke" your eyes, just apply eye shadow in a similar shade over the liner. If the liner smudges, clean up with a slightly dampened cotton swab.

Wide Eyes

Apply a shimmery beige shadow from lash line to brow bone. Finish with a slightly darker shadow on the lids for definition.

Expert Eyes

You can actually change the shape of your eyes with the right makeup techniques.

No matter the size or shape of your eyes,

you can make your eyes bigger, wider, and more dramatic.

Small Eyes

Use pale and medium shadows, and stay away from dark colors or dark eyeliner. Apply light shadow over the lids, and a line of medium shadow in the crease.

Close-Set Eyes

You can visually separate close-set eyes by using light, shimmery shades at the inner corner of each eye. It gives the illusion of more space. Line the outer half of the eye with darker shadow.

Deep-Set Eyes

Deep-set eyes need to come out of hiding. Use a pale shadow all over the lid, and only the lid. Line with a pale liner, and smudge the two together.

Wide-Set Eyes

Wide set eyes come together by applying dark color at the inner corner of each eye. Apply a lighter shadow at the outer corners.

SHADOW TRICK

Use your fingertip to blend your eye shadow. Take what's left on your finger and press against the outer, lower rim.

GREAT LIPS

PLUMPER LIPS WITHOUT COLLAGEN

No, you don't have to spend a ton of money keeping up those collagen treatments. Cinnamon oil plumps up your lips by increasing blood flow to the lips.

As a bonus, it leaves lips with a slight rosy tint. You'll find cinnamon oil at natural supermarkets and health food stores. Make sure you test it on your wrist to ensure that you aren't sensitive or allergic to the oil.

WHAT COLOR?

Fair complexions: pale pink, beige, or cool red
Medium: Burgundy, caramel, or berry

Olive/Yellow: brown and plums

Dark: Berry, dark red, beige

WHAT KIND?

It's confusing to decide what lipstick to get when there are so many types. Each has its unique qualities and advantages.

Long-wearing: Stays for four to five hours, but can also feel dry.

Transfer-resistant: Lasts up to eight hours, but can make lips dry and may be hard to remove.

Matte: Lots of color, but can look dull.

Cream: Contains lighter waxes, but needs reapplication.

Moisturizing: Makes lips soft and shiny, but doesn't last.

Satin: Lots of oil and moisturizing, but looks darker than actual color.

Get Smooth

Before you apply your lipstick, make sure your lips are soft and flake-free. Brush your teeth, and then gently brush your lips to remove dead skin. Coat lips with a lip balm and allow it to soak in while you do the rest of your makeup.

MAKE small LIPS LOOK FULLER

- Stay away from very dark colors. Deep shades make thin lips look hard and small.
- Using a neutral lip pencil, draw slightly outside the line.
- Go for a little shimmer. A light-reflective surface can make your lips appear larger. Don't use too much since gloss reflects light and can make lips fade.

LIP TRICKS

- Open your mouth when applying your lipstick.

- Use a nude, never a colored, lipliner.

- Create a fuller-looking mouth by putting a spot of light-weight concealer on the center of your lips after applying lipstick. Then lightly blend it out toward the corners.

- Apply lip pencil along the Cupid's bow of your upper lip.

- Never go over your natural lip line.

Apply lip balm, then **BLOT** excess off with a tissue. Line the outer lip with a pencil that matches the balm, then pencil in. **BLOT** again to blend.

MAKE **FULL** LIPS LOOK s m a l l e r

• Play up your eyes.
• Use a neutral colored lipstick.
• Don't bother with a lipliner.
• Apply lipstick right from the tube and blend.
• Blot so there's only pigment left on the lips.
• Since you don't need to define your lips, go for blurred borders.

ADD SOME **CURVES**

Using a pencil the color of your lips, draw a V in the bow area of your upper lip, going just above your natural lip line.

FIX IT **FAST**

Tone down that too-bright lipstick by mixing a small dab of foundation with petroleum jelly and patting it over lips.

INSTEAD OF LINER

Get a line around your lips without bothering with lipliner by applying your lipstick with a brush.

TIME SAVER

Dip a lip pencil in lip gloss and apply all over lips. The gloss will soften the pencil so that it spreads smoothly.

The **GREASIER** the lipstick, the more it **BLEEDS**. Brown pigments need more oils, so brown lipsticks will probably be greasier.

TESTING LIPSTICK

You probably think that the correct way to test lipstick is on the back of your hand. But makeup artists know that the true color will come out on your fingertips. The texture and color of the skin on your fingers is more like your lips.

BLUSH

Here's the #1 Rule: The brighter the blush, the less area it should cover. When using a bright shade, use it only on the apples of your cheeks.

Pink is most flattering to very pale skin.

Medium skin should lean toward darker pink or light bronze.

Yellow tones will find that berries and plums will counteract sallowness.

Ethnic skins can still wear pink, but a slightly browner tone.

CONTOURING

With the right contouring techniques, it can look like you've lost weight, you've changed the shape of your face, and you've got the planes and angles of a top supermodel.

When you try to contour and you do it incorrectly, it ends up looking like you've got streaks of dirt on your face.

Choose a color tone. Contouring can help create shadows where they don't normally occur. Go no more than two shades deeper than your natural skin tone. Otherwise it makes your face look strange.

Apply color by sucking in your cheeks, and with your fingers, feel your cheekbones. Step your fingers down until you feel natural hollows. This is the area where you should concentrate your blush. Roll the brush up to your temples. Don't just sweep it up, or it will give you a line. Lightly rolling will appear more natural.

Right above your blush, apply a highlighter. Be sure to blend the edges with the blush with your fingers. The goal is to never let any lines show on your face.

Long Face

Dust blush on top of your forehead, along your jawline, and under your cheekbones. Don't go too far down your face, no farther than the bottom of your nose.

Square Face

Shade the sides of your jaw and forehead. Sweep over your cheekbones

Heart-Shaped Face

Shade the sides of your forehead, temples, and tip of your chin. Sweep over your cheekbones.

MAKEUP PRO RULES

- Always apply cream products before powder.
- Dot dark eye pencil or liner between lashes to give the appearance of thicker lashes.
- Shorten your nose with bronzing powder or a darker foundation at the tip.

SLIM YOUR NOSE by applying a stripe of lighter powder or foundation down the center of your nose.

Never apply concealer around the eye area without eye cream. The dryness and thickness of the concealer will make skin look cracked.

Pencil needs to be sealed. Otherwise it will smear and disappear. Apply similarly colored shadow over it.

Eye shadow needs to be primed with powder. Otherwise it will crease.

Apply lipliner after lipstick. In this way you can see where you need to correct.

Make your eye shadow **LAST ALL DAY** by applying foundation on lids with a makeup sponge or your fingers. Pat gently, creating a surface for the shadow to hold on to.

MONEY SAVING ADVICE

Always CLOSE THE LIDS of all your cosmetics. Allowing air to get in will SHORTEN the effectiveness of any product and its shelf life.

NO LONGER A BARGAIN

If there is any kind of SMELL or other ODOR coming from any beauty product, IT'S GONE BAD. Throw it away immediately.

COMMON MAKEUP MISTAKES

DON'T

- Close your eyes while applying eyeliner
- Forget to blend each product
- Sharpen your pencils so much that it creates an obvious line
- Match your eye products to your clothing
- Try to get cheekbones with blush
- Attempt to make your face brighter with your foundation

DO

- Lift your chin and look down into a mirror when applying eye products
- Blot your entire face with a separated tissue
- Roll hard pencil tips between your fingers to soften.
- Use a slightly darker foundation color to contour

Chapter 11

HAIR BARGAINS

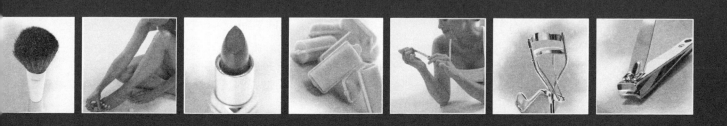

CHEAP CHANGES

Your hair is an inexpensive way to change your looks.

You don't need to spend a lot on hair products to have great hair. You'll find very good shampoos, conditioners, brushes, rollers, and just about any other styling product you can think of at drugstores and discount stores.

WORTH THE COST

The better the haircut, the easier the upkeep. A good cut will allow you to go through the day, the weather, whatever happens, and it can still look good. If you need to choose when to spend on your hair, splurge on a good haircut.

WORK WITH WHAT YOU'VE GOT

If you've been blessed with incredible curls, don't get too hung up on keeping them stick-straight no matter what the current trend. Be brave. One day when you can relax and when you don't have to have any important pictures taken, let your hair dry naturally. You may be pleasantly surprised.

YOU JUST NEED A FEW TOOLS

The right tools create the right look You only need a couple of essentials. It's how they're made, not how much you've spent.

A GOOD BRUSH

A natural bristle like boar's hair is worth the purchase. Animal bristles are like your hair. They're porous, and help lift the natural oils from your scalp and spread them throughout your hair. In this way, your hair oils will be distributed throughout and will provide shine.

Choose a synthetic brush if your hair is very thick and tends to tangle. Synthetic bristles are usually made of nylon and are stronger, which makes them more effective at getting rid of knots and taming unruly hair.

If you have a lot of highlights, consider a metal brush to keep the shine. Metal brushes act like flatirons to seal the cuticle.

For smoothing, an oversized paddle brush is perfect. It helps hair fall smooth. A paddle brush is also good for drying long hair because it grabs many strands of hair at a time.

HAIR DRYER

Choose one that's comfortable to hold, with enough heat to seal the cuticle. A hair dryer with 1875 watts is a good value. Different speeds are a good option.

Look for the "cool shot" feature. It's a button that lets you blast your locks with cold air to seal the cuticle and get rid of frizz. It also helps boost shine.

CHOOSE YOUR PRODUCTS CAREFULLY

It's always important to check the labels of your hair products. Certain ingredients will provide certain results.

If you want great gloss, check the labels for products containing jojoba or aloe. These ingredients are effective at providing shine without grease.

To get your hair straight, look for citrus ingredients. Products should contain ingredients like grapefruit, orange, and lime. They help straighten hair and help to prevent waving caused by moisture.

DON'T **WASTE** YOUR MONEY

CHEAP SHAMPOO washes excess product from the hair and scalp better than any of the expensive brands. **POMADES** are pretty much all the same. Drugstores sell great ones like Murray's.

You don't need a lot of different products. A little **STYLING LOTION** will both add **SHINE AND HOLD** to your hair.

To increase volume in your hair, look for ingredients like polymers. These are synthetic molecules that expand the natural space between hairs to give strands extra lift.

To fight frizz, products should contain proteins, which help stabilize the natural proteins in your own hair.

To soften hair, your product should contain silicone. This helps to strengthen and moisturize hair as well as protect it from styling products that use heat.

HAIR COLOR

Maybe you were born with beautiful light blonde hair, but all of a sudden puberty hit, and your color is starting to turn a dull brown. Or you never liked your color, and you want a change. There are lots of ways to make fun changes.

SEMI PERMANENT DYE

It's a good way to experiment, because if you don't like it, it won't damage your hair, and you won't be stuck with it.

HIGHLIGHTS

If you can afford it, try having a professional do this for you. If you can't, then ask a friend. Adding a few streaks to your hair is a fun way to get started. Plus, there are several "at home" coloring kits that are inexpensive and have really complete instructions.

WASH-OUT COLOR

These last about four weeks, and can help you decide if you're really meant to be a redhead.

WIG OUT!

It's a painless way to see if you like that hair color. It's also a great preview to a new hairstyle.

COLORING TIPS

- The ends of your hair are more porous and soak up more color than the roots. Rub conditioner over the ends while your hair is processing. In the last five minutes, apply color to the ends, over the conditioner. The color will penetrate just enough to create an even color.

Shampoo your hair THE DAY BEFORE you color it. That way, you will be less likely to have streaks.

If your shampoo doesn't lather very much, it's LOW pH.

- For root touch-ups (and nothing else), part your hair into four equal sections. Keep the sections in place with bobby pins or clips. Apply the color to the parts themselves. Take each section and work on the roots of the section, and then clip up again. This keeps the coloring on the root, and keeps you from wasting product.
- Use a shampoo with a low pH level so that it won't strip out your color.
- Spread petroleum jelly along hairline before applying color to protect your skin.
- Peroxide-based astringents like Sea Breeze can give very subtle highlights. Use a toothbrush and simply apply product to thin sections of hair. Let it sit ten minutes and shampoo thoroughly.
- Try to find products with thermal protectors. These products have barriers to protect hair from heat.

- Always rinse with cool water after every wash to extend the life of your color.

COLORING MYTH

Some women think that their color will not get as dark as it is shown on the box if they leave it on five or so minutes less than directed. That isn't enough time for the color to take and the results leave the hair looking brassy.

HAIR SEASONS

SUMMER

- Heat proof your hair and stop your color from fading.

- Make sure your product has UV filters.
- Wear a hat.
- Use a color-protecting shampoo.
- After swimming in the pool, rinse your hair in apple cider vinegar to remove the chlorine.

STEAMY SCALP.

USE A **MINT SHAMPOO OR CONDITIONER**. IT WILL ACTUALLY LOWER THE SCALP'S TEMPERATURE.

SUMMER STYLE

Here is the perfect summer hairdo. Before you head to the beach, braid your hair. After going into the water, unravel the braids. Your hair will look hot-rollered. Plus, you'll get great texture because the salt makes the hair extra scrunchable.

You can get the same look without the ocean by combining one-third cup of salt with two-thirds cup of water in a spray bottle and spritzing all over hair.

You can use the sun to highlight your hair. Put on a straw hat and pull random strands of hair through the holes. For the most natural look, concentrate on pieces around your face. Spritz exposed hair with fresh lemon juice in a spray bottle and let the rays do their work. The juice should dry. Use a deep conditioner after this treatment.

WINTER

- If your hair is covered with snow, don't comb it out until it dries.
- Shake the excess water and snow out.
- If your hair has frozen (it can happen!), thaw it out with a hair dryer set on low.
- Protect your hair with a good silicone finishing treatment.

PRO SECRETS

FIGHT **FRIZZ**

Just spritz damp hair with a light conditioning spray. Then let your hair air dry, or blow it dry on low or with a diffuser.

COWLICK CONTROL

After you've styled your hair, wet the cowlick and position it in place. Keep it there with a wax or pomade.

HEALTHY HAIR

Use a nourishing mask at least once a week. You'll find them in drugstores with names like "deep treatment."

BED HEAD

Love that look that you've seen on the runways? Vary the amount of styling cream you use all over your head. It will create a multi-textured effect.

CONTROL YOUR CURLS

Use a heated comb. Set it on low to medium and run it over any area that you need to smooth.

HAVE A **TRIM**

Even if you are trying to grow your hair out, you need to have your hair trimmed every four to six weeks. It will get rid of dead split ends and will even help your hair grow faster.

A hot oil treatment makes your hair shiny and manageable. Just use olive oil. Warm it up and coat your dry, unwashed hair with it. Sit out in the sun for twenty minutes. Wash it out thoroughly and condition.

GREAT HAIR ON A BUDGET

USE **COLD** WATER

Make your final rinse a cold one. It will really make your hair shine.

DETOX YOUR PRODUCTS

Add a couple of aspirin to your shampoo to take out the entire excess product and get your hair squeaky clean.

GET RID OF **OIL**

Dip your fingers in baking soda and massage your scalp to instantly dry up oil. It's a great way to revive your style.

LEND A **HAND**

If you want to tame flyaways and give your hair a little shine, run some hand lotion over it. Just rub the lotion in the palms of your hands, and then run your palms over your hair. Don't use too much lotion or it will look greasy.

HAIR ACCESSORIES ON THE CHEAP

Recycle your panty hose and make your own scrunchies.
Cut your hose in three- to four-inch lengths. You'll love the way you can match your hair color, and your hair will not be snagged or pulled as with an elastic band.

RECYCLE YOUR OLD JEWELRY

Rings can dress up hair ties.

Pins can become great barrettes with a bobby pin or two.

A necklace turns into a creative headband.

Clip on earrings make great hair accents.

Be creative and have fun!

HAIR EMERGENCIES

How do you solve that hair problem? You do it quickly and creatively. Here are some of my favorites.

HAIR IS **TOTALLY TANGLED**

Dampen hair and then straighten out starting from the ends.

FLAT HAIR

Blow hair out straight and then set it for a few minutes on hot rollers to give it more volume.

Revive your hair in the shower. Pull your hair into a ponytail on top of your head, separate into two sections and wrap two them around Velcro rollers. Cover with a shower cap. The steam will help set your hair and give it volume and curves by the time you get out.

NO TIME TO SHAMPOO

When you don't have time to wash your hair, mist it with an aerosol hair spray. Then run your fingers through. The alcohol will dissolve the oil and revive your style. If there's no hair spray on hand, use perfume. There's enough alcohol in the fragrance to give your style new life.

BANGS ARE **TOO LONG**

Dampen your hair and comb forward the bangs that go from the middle on one eyebrow to the center of the other. Pull tight and cut right at the bridge of your nose. Your bangs will pop back up to your brows in a natural line.

ROOTS ARE SHOWING

- Make a zig-zag part.
- Cover your roots with chalk. Washable magic marker also works in a pinch.
- Eye shadow can be blended for a perfect match. Apply it with your fingers or a small sponge-tipped applicator.
- Paint roots away with washable mascara.

LAYERS ARE **GROWING OUT**

Use the top layers you're trying to grow out to create extra volume. After drying, spritz roots at the crown with spray gel. Tease a bit to create fullness.

Control layers by applying a super hold gel to damp hair then combing through. Secure layers with a clip and allow hair to air dry.

ENDS ARE **UNEVEN**

Blow dry while using a round brush to flip ends up. For extra hold, blow dry with cool air and spritz with hair spray.

Rub hair wax on ends and heat with a blow dryer. The ends will fuse together temporarily.

TOO MUCH OIL

The pectin in apple juice absorbs excess oil, leaving hair squeaky clean. In a pitcher, combine one-third cup apple juice with one-half teaspoon white vinegar, which intensifies the juices and has oil-absorbing power. Pour over freshly washed hair. Comb through; and leave on for fifteen minutes. Rinse and follow with a light shampoo.

IN NEED OF **GREASE RELIEF**

Make several parts in your hair around the crown. Apply witch hazel with a cotton ball. Stroke over your scalp. This treatment also helps to control dandruff.

DANDRUFF DUTY

Lemon is a natural exfoliant that fights dandruff. Spritz hair with the juice of one lemon mixed with two cups water. Then shampoo. Rinse with two teaspoons lemon and one cup cool water.

STOP **BREAKAGE**

Stop hair brittleness and breakage with soy milk. It nourishes the cuticle to restore strength and flexibility. Combine one-half cup soy milk and three tablespoons of cornstarch. Comb through wet hair and let stand ten minutes. Rinse well.

SPECIALTY TREATMENTS

BLACK TEA TONIC

Black tea is good for your hair, too.

Add two tablespoons of dried rosemary to two cups of brewed tea.

Let steep for ten minutes

Pour the mixture over your head and massage for one minute. Rinse thoroughly.

APPLE CIDER SHAMPOO

Combine equal amounts of apple cider vinegar and shampoo in a clean container.

Shake well to blend.

This shampoo will get rid of residue and buildup.

RHUBARB HIGHLIGHTS

Add one-quarter cup of chopped fresh rhubarb to two cups of boiling water. Let the mixture cool and strain through a sieve. Work it through your hair after shampooing, then rinse.

PEAR PACK

Pears are great for providing incredible texture and volume. Run a ripe Bosc pear under warm water to soften. Canned pears can also be used with no need to soften. Peel and remove seeds. Place the pear in a bowl and mash with a fork. Mix in one teaspoon plain gelatin. Apply the mixture to just-washed hair, massaging into the scalp and working throughout. Leave on for fifteen minutes and then shampoo out.

A **GRAPEFRUIT'S** high acidity stabilizes the hair's pH level, keeping the cuticle sleek and smooth. Add a **HALF A CUP** of juice to your shampoo.

Honey Maple Treatment

This is the cheapest and most intense treatment for damaged hair that you can make.

one teaspoon **canola oil**

one teaspoon **softened margarine**

one teaspoon **maple syrup**

one teaspoon **honey**

- HEAT above in microwave until warm

- MASSAGE mixture through hair

- Let SET fifteen minutes

- RINSE and then SHAMPOO

"ADULTS ONLY" HAIR TREATMENTS

Fun with Beer

Not only can beer liven up a dull party, it can also give life to your hair.

Microwave a cup of flat beer for sixty seconds. This removes the alcohol that can dry hair. Let the beer cool and mix it with your favorite shampoo. The hops make your hair more shiny and radiant

Crack open a cold one and pour over towel-dried hair. Let sit for five minutes and then rinse with cool water. This treatment makes hair glossy and thick, and no, you won't smell like a brewery.

Combine a cup of ale with three cups water, and pour over freshly washed hair. Comb through. Wait three minutes and rinse. Follow with conditioner.

Va Va Vodka

Combine one tablespoon of vodka with half a cup of seltzer. The bubbles in alcohol cut through product buildup to give hair super shine. Use as a final rinse after washing hair.

Mix one-quarter cup of vodka with one-quarter cup of shampoo for a shine-producing, clarifying shampoo.

Champagne Chunks

Bring out your highlights by combining one-half cup of champagne with one-half cup of shampoo. Follow with your regular conditioner.

Tropical Rum Conditioner

This is an excellent conditioner for dry, damaged hair. Mix together one egg with three tablespoons rum. Pour mixture on hair and let set two to three minutes. Rinse well with cool water for extra shine.

HOW HEALTHY IS YOUR HAIR?

Use a mirror to look at the back of your hair inside a brightly lit room. You should be able to see a shine line surrounding your hair like a halo: otherwise, you're missing shine. Excessive blow-drying, frequent coloring, and even your hormones can increase pH levels in your hair, causing dullness. Reflect more light by using a lower pH shampoo. It will be listed on the bottle.

Healthy hair is soft. Measure hair softness by running your fingers through your hair from roots to the ends of the hair. It should feel fully silky, and should glide through your fingers easily. Otherwise you need to deep condition.

Healthy hair is elastic and strong. Test yours by stretching a strand from the scalp. If your hair can stretch significantly without snapping then it's strong.

FREEBIE

Shampoos containing silicones can help with hair strength. Also be sure to get enough protein in your diet.

HAIR TRADITION

For centuries, women have poured olive oil over their hair as a beauty treatment. And now all the top hair products being sold are featuring olive oil. You can have the same effect by using olive oil straight from the bottle. You'll save lots of money and your hair will look better than ever.

Heat for a second or two in the microwave and apply to hair before shampooing. Massage a few drops in the palms of your hands and run over dry hair to refresh.

Get your hair glowing and your frustrations out!

Beat a handful of papaya leaves in a bucket of water until you create a lather. Use this as a conditioner after shampooing.

COPY THIS STYLIST SECRET.
After shampooing, finish with a blast of cool water. It feeds the hair cuticle to make your hair shine.

NIGHT WORK

How you style your hair at night can make a big difference between bed head and ready to go.

- If you have long hair, secure it loosely in a big ponytail.

- If your hair is cut in layers, wrap sections around your finger and secure with bobby pins. You'll wake up with loose, sexy waves.

- If you have short or medium hair, keep it smooth by wearing a wide cloth headband. When it comes off, you'll have lots of volume.

TIME SAVERS

- If your hair is straight, finger comb only until it's at least 80 percent dry.
- If your hair is wavy, wrap your wet hair in a moisture-absorbing towel for about twenty minutes.
- If your hair is curly, wash and air-dry your hair.

THE PERFECT CUT

Show your stylist exactly where you want your hair to fall rather than telling her you just want her to cut an inch. It's the only time when it's perfectly polite to point.

Get the cut you really want by bringing your hair dresser a picture. It says a thousand words. Have you ever tried to explain a haircut you've seen? It's not possible.

Keep it simple: the most elegant haircut is above the shoulders with a few angled layers in front.

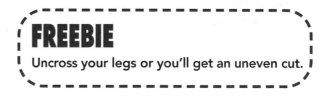

FREEBIE
Uncross your legs or you'll get an uneven cut.

Chapter 12

HEAVENLY HANDS

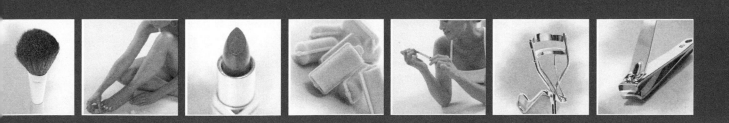

They're constantly on display. Your hands are an expression of your style and your attention to detail. The good news is that it doesn't cost a lot to keep them looking great once you learn to do it yourself.

PERFECT NAILS

POLISH POINTERS

Avoid quick-drying polishes. They have a large amount of acetone, which dries out polish and causes cracks. Use regular polishes instead for a manicure that will last three times longer.

FREEBIE
Store polish in the refrigerator for a longer life.

Prevent bubbles by prepping nails with witch hazel.

Always roll, never shake the bottle, or you're sure to get bubbles. Just roll the bottle between your palms. That's more than enough to thoroughly mix polish.

Dip nails in ice water for ten seconds to set color.

The very same shine serum that you use on your hair can make your nails look kept and your polish look brand-new. Place a couple of drops on a cotton ball and buff nails until shiny.

To keep polish from bleeding into the cracks, apply cuticle oil to the surrounding skin before you apply color. Then it's easy to wipe off excess after polishing.

Always make sure that each polish coat is as thin as possible. Thicker coats don't dry enough between coats to adhere to nail properly and so polish will peel off more easily.

Always use polish thinner, not polish remover, to extend the life of your old polish.

REMOVE POLISH STAINS

- Soak nails in white vinegar for ten minutes.
- Add two teaspoons of household bleach to one-half cup of warm water and soak nails for fifteen minutes.

IF NAILS ARE LONGER THAN ONE EIGHTH OF AN INCH, THEY SHOULD BE CLIPPED BEFORE FILING. OTHERWISE, JUST FILE.

MAKE YOUR MANICURE LAST

- Buff before polishing to smooth down the nail surface.
- Make sure your nails are totally dry before applying polish.
- Never soak nails before applying polish. The moisture will remain and causes the polish to lift.

FREEBIE

One coat is all you need of light polish. Most darker colors require at least two coats.

DO-IT-YOURSELF **FRENCH MANICURE**

The French manicure is one of the most sought-after looks. It looks natural and fresh, and if done right, very classy. It also costs a lot to have it done professionally, and just as much for the upkeep. In just five easy steps, and in just minutes, you can give yourself a professional-looking French manicure. Don't worry if you don't get it perfect the first time. Just keep at it. You'll soon become an expert.

1. Apply a basecoat over clean, buffed nails.

2. Follow with one or two coats of natural pink or nude color polish.

3. Holding the end of a nail file almost to the edge of your nail, sweep a line of white polish across the entire tip. Try to do it in one stroke.

4. Follow up with another coat of your first polish, covering the entire nail, including the white edge.

5. Finish with a topcoat to provide shine and protection.

NAIL ART

- Glue a charm to the nail when polish starts to set.
- Follow with clear polish to help it stick.

PROBLEM SOLVING YOUR NAILS

STAINS

Not only are dark polishes the cause of stained nails, but nicotine and certain foods can do it, too. Rub a slice of fresh lemon over nails or try a cotton swab dipped in hydrogen peroxide. My favorite treatment is using two denture cleanser tablets in a cup of water and letting my nails soak for a few minutes.

NAIL SPLITTING

In some cases, brittle nails can be caused by protein or vitamin deficiencies. Consider taking vitamin B or silica tablets. Check with your doctor first and make sure to apply a nail hardener daily. The hardener is not going to make your nails grow faster or grow stronger, but it does form a protective barrier.

NAIL HARDENERS

Are your nails constantly chipping, peeling, and breaking? Look no further than these fast fixes.

1. Massage garlic oil into the nail bed and cuticle.
2. Look for a nail hardener with calcium. Don't forget to apply under nails, too.
3. Rub hair conditioner into your nails. It contains proteins to strengthen nails.

If you have spent a lot of money on nail strengtheners but are still left with **SOFT, PEELING NAILS,** it could be caused by your face moisturizer. If it contains glycolic acid, it has the ability to exfoliate and get under the nails, causing them to split. Wash your hands immediately after applying your cream.

CUTICLE CARE

After cuticles have soaked, push them back gently. Brush away stray pieces of dead skin with a buffing disk.

BRIGHTEN NAILS

Fill a bowl with warm water. Add one-half teaspoon of sea salt and one sliced lime. Soak hands for ten minutes.

Mix one tablespoon of hydrogen peroxide with two tablespoons of baking soda. Brush on nails with a small toothbrush. Rinse immediately.

Dip a nailbrush into equal parts lemon juice, white vinegar, and water. The water should be warm. Brush over stained or yellowed nails, wait a few seconds, then rinse.

IF YOU'RE REALLY ON THE RUN, HERE'S AN INSTANT FIX THAT WILL ALSO SOFTEN YOUR CUTICLES.

Rub a drop of **olive oil** to each nail to revive the topcoat's sheen.

CITRUS CUTICLE **SMOOTHER**

Soak fingertips in one cup warm water combined with the juice of a lemon. After five minutes, the citric acid will soften ragged, hard cuticles so that you can push them back with a cloth.

REMOVE **EXCESS** CUTICLE

Scrub excess cuticle away with toothpaste. It works to soften and get rid of ragged edges.

Smooth the skin by rubbing petroleum jelly or bag balm (available in the skincare section of most drugstores) to lock in moisture and soften rough edges.

HEAL **RAGGED** CUTICLES

For a freshly manicured look, combine a bottle of cuticle oil with a cup of hot water. Wait sixty seconds, and then brush over your cuticles. The water and the oil combine to provide instantly smoother cuticles.

SUPPLE SKIN

Consider vitamin C cream to keep your hands wrinkle-free. Vitamin C has the ability to restore softness and boost collagen production.

Massage hands and feet with an alpha hydroxy lotion. Before doing so, coat nails with lip balm to prevent breakage and splitting.

Apply moisturizer before you put on your rubber gloves to wash dishes. It will make the cream really work.

HAND **SOFTENER**

Warm a cup of olive oil in the microwave for ten seconds in a small microwaveable bowl. Make sure the oil is comfortable to the touch (after heating). Soak hands for ten to fifteen minutes. Rinse and pat dry.

LEMON HAND **HEALER**

This lemon paste penetrates and heals dry skin. Mix one tablespoon of lemon juice, one tablespoon of honey, and one-quarter cup of olive oil. Massage as a paste over clean hands and cover with a plastic bag for twenty minutes. Rinse well.

PAMPERING PARAFFIN

Drown your hands in moisture by giving them a paraffin wax treatment. You can find paraffin bars at supermarkets, or you can use old candles. Simply put them in the microwave until they melt. First apply a thin layer of vegetable oil on hands and then dip into warm, never hot, wax. Allow to harden, and then peel off.

HAND REVIVER

Soak your hands in a combination of two teaspoons of baking soda and one denture cleanser tablet in a small bowl of warm water for five minutes. This solution will wake up your fingers and clean your nails. Complete the treatment by rubbing your favorite cleanser into the tops of hands around nails and cuticles with a vegetable brush. Rinse and pat dry.

PRO TREATMENT

Warm moisturizer in microwave for about ten seconds or until just warm. Rub into hands and feet. Slip on cotton gloves and cotton socks for added benefits. Let the cream do its work for about fifteen minutes, and then rinse off.

Chapter 13

FABULOUS FEET

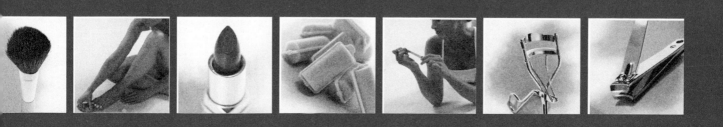

SOFTEN THAT SKIN

Fill a basin with warm water and add the juice of a lemon with one cup of oatmeal. Soak feet for ten minutes. While soaking, rub the oatmeal all over your feet. The oatmeal will soften rough feet while the lemon will lighten and even out skin.

File rough spots with a coarse nail file.

Combine one-half cup of sugar, one-quarter teaspoon of poppy seeds, and one-quarter baking soda with a few drops of lemon juice. Scrub briskly with a vegetable brush and rinse thoroughly.

Apply **Vicks VapoRub** on dry feet before bed. Wear socks, and your feet will be smooth and silky the next morning.

FOOT MASSAGE

Apply any oil, and gently rub the tops, sides, and bottoms of your feet in circular movements using both your thumbs and fingers.

FOOT TONIC

Microwave the following:

One cup milk

One tablespoon dry mint leaves

1 tsp. rosemary

1 tsp. peppermint extract

Apply the mixture to feet with a clean, dry cloth. Remove residue and wrap feet in plastic wrap. Wait five minutes and rinse thoroughly.

THE PERFECT PEDICURE

1. File nails straight across. You don't want to risk ingrown toenails or weaken your nails.
2. Remove moisture by swiping rubbing alcohol over the nail bed.
3. Push back cuticles.
4. Prep with a base coat. Place tissues between toes to prevent smearing.
5. Apply polish starting with the smallest toe of the hand you don't write with.
6. Apply two coats, waiting five minutes in between coats.
7. Wait five minutes more, and then apply topcoat.
8. Erase any mistakes with a cotton swab dipped in polish remover.

PLEASE DON'T !

Wear OPEN-TOED SHOES or SANDALS without manicured feet. Even if you like your nails natural, you still need a gloss over them to protect and strengthen them.

PEDICURE RULES

- Start with soft skin.
- Smoothe any and all ridges.
- Never apply lotion between toes because moisture there can lead to skin fungus.
- Don't shave off calluses and corns with a razor. Just put a little muscle into your nail file.
- Always wait an hour before putting shoes back on.

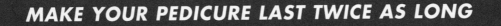

MAKE YOUR PEDICURE LAST TWICE AS LONG

1. Choose metallic or shimmery polishes. They contain minerals that adhere to the nail better and cause it to last much longer.

2. Brush on several thin coats rather than one thick layer.

3. Wait five minutes before applying the topcoat. If the polish hasn't set, it will thin out and be more prone to chipping.

KEEP YOUR FEET SWEET

Make sure your footwear fits properly. Your socks need room for your toes to wiggle.

To protect feet from new shoe friction, dab sensitive areas with petroleum jelly. Or apply a small patch of adhesive moleskin, which you can get at most drugstores.

FOOT EXERCISE

Rub your foot over a soda can or a tennis ball to help cramps and to relax feet.

FOOT REFRESHER

The perfect way to refresh feet after a long day at the office: add six drops of both eucalyptus and rosemary oil to a pan of hot water. Soak for about ten minutes. Rinse, alternating between hot and cold water to improve circulation.

SHOE SUPPORT

Sneakers are a great bargain, but you need to replace them every four to six months. Wear and tear breaks them down on the inside and subsequently takes away the support that you need.

Try on sneakers in the late afternoon when feet have swollen.

HAVE BOTH FEET MEASURED EACH TIME YOU SHOP FOR SNEAKERS OR SHOES BECAUSE FOOT SIZE INCREASES WITH AGE, WEIGHT, AND PREGNANCY.

Make sure the widest part of your foot fits comfortably within the widest part of the shoe.

Look for a roomy toe box that will allow you to wiggle all your toes.

Your feet should feel snug and not slip when you walk.

Flex sneaker soles between the heel and toe area to be sure that they are flexible, but not too flexible. If it's too flexible, then the front will touch the heel with virtually no stress. It's too rigid if it is almost impossible to bend.

Most importantly, the sneaker should be comfortable right out of the box. Walk around for a few minutes to make sure you could walk in the shoes all day.

SOOTHE ACHING FEET

Combine a teaspoon of coconut oil and five drops of rosemary essential oil in a microwave-safe container. Heat until coconut oil is melted, about five or six seconds. Fill a small basin halfway with warm water and add the mixture. Soak about fifteen minutes and pat dry.

GET RID OF CORNS

Soak your feet in warm salt water. Buff the affected area with a coarse emery board. Apply a pineapple slice for five minutes over the corn. The enzymes will further dissolve the corn. Rub in lotion and sleep wearing socks.

Replace plastic heel tips with rubber for comfort and safety.

Chapter 14

SPA SAVINGS

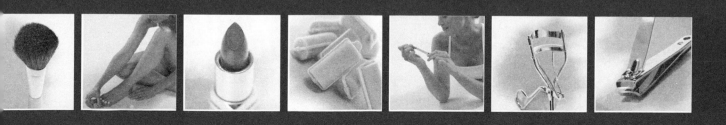

You can easily replicate at home the very treatments you could spend a fortune on in spas. After all, spas pride themselves on homeopathic, fresh ingredients in their concoctions. I've spent years uncovering their secrets, and I'm so happy to be able to pass them along.

ACNE TREATMENTS

BLEMISH BUSTING MASK

Mix one-half teaspoon turmeric with enough water to form a paste. Apply to blemishes, and leave on overnight.

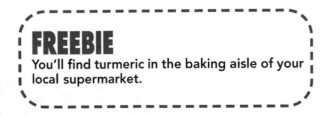

FREEBIE
You'll find turmeric in the baking aisle of your local supermarket.

SOOTHE INFLAMED SKIN WITH WITCH HAZEL.

HONEY/ORANGE 5-MINUTE MASK

Apply one-half cup honey with one-half cup orange juice to blemishes. Leave on five minutes before rinsing. The honey contains hydrogen peroxide, which inhibits bacteria, while the citric acid in the juice will dry up excess oil.

Wash acne-prone areas with a little **tea tree oil** mixed with an equal amount of warm water.

BLACKHEAD REMOVER

Here's a way to get rid of blackheads naturally (and without squeezing!). Dissolve one tablespoon of unflavored gelatin in two tablespoons of milk over low heat. Let cool and apply to face. Leave on thirty minutes. As you peel off the mask, you'll peel off the blackheads.

COMPLEXION-CORRECTING FACIAL

This two-step process has two wonderful ingredients. The banana is full of vitamin B to nourish your skin, while the egg white will absorb oil.

Step 1

Mix together one teaspoon of honey with one egg white, and apply to face. Allow to dry and rinse.

Step 2

Mash one banana with a tablespoon of avocado. Leave on for ten minutes and rinse.

CHAMOMILE COMPLEXION CALMER

Mix one-half cup of powdered chamomile with enough water to make a thick paste. You'll find powdered chamomile at health food stores. Spread over entire face, avoiding the eye area, and allow to set for five minutes. Rinse with cool water.

SPA EXFOLIATORS

- Powdered milk with water is a clean and natural milk cleanser. Plus it's convenient since you don't have to refrigerate it.
- Salt is good for chafed skin or for removing a peeling sunburn. Mix a one-half teaspoon salt with a teaspoon of water.
- Baking soda with water is a good wash for very sensitive skin. Put a little baking soda in the palm of your hand, and then add just enough water to make a paste.

PAPAYA ENZYME TREATMENT

This treatment may take more time than most but is highly effective in clearing up blemishes.

MASH a very ripe papaya into a pulp.

BOIL two quarts of water with a packet of an herbal laxative.

APPLY mashed papaya to your face (avoiding eye area).

KEEP your face over the steaming water (keeping a comfortable distance).

PUT a towel over your head to direct the steam to your face.

DO this for about ten minutes.

RINSE with warm water and gently pat dry.

INSTANT SKIN REVIVER

Squeeze an orange and pat the liquid on your face with your fingers. The citrus liquid and scent will evaporate quickly, but you'll look awesome. It's all thanks to the vitamin C, an antioxidant that gives a great glow.

CHEAP & EFFECTIVE

Moisturize your body

with a vegetable

shortening like Crisco.

Moisturize your face only if it's extremely dry or sunburned.

YUMMY MASKS AND WRAPS

AVOCADO FACE MASK

Mash a teaspoon of ripe avocado with one-half teaspoon of lemon juice. Massage into face and neck. Let dry, and then rinse off with cool water.

COGNAC MASK

A spa owner attributes this facial treatment to Marie Antoinette, who was legendary for her glowing and flawless skin.

Combine one tablespoon of cognac with a whole egg, one-quarter cup of milk powder, and the juice of a lemon. Apply all over face and allow to dry. Rinse off thoroughly with tepid water.

131

ALOE VERA MASK

Here is a treatment that produces a cool soothing effect while toning the skin.

Mix one-quarter cup of aloe vera gel with the contents of two capsules pure vitamin E. Add one-half teaspoon of tea tree oil with the leafy contents of one slightly steeped chamomile tea bag. Let set for thirty minutes to one hour. Apply to clean face using upward strokes and avoiding the eyes. Allow to warm on face for fifteen minutes and then rinse off with cold water.

BEFORE BATHING OR SHOWERING, BRUSH YOUR BODY WITH AN EXFOLIATING BATH BRUSH. IT'S USED IN SPAS TO BOOST CIRCULATION, DELIVERING MORE OXYGEN AND NUTRIENTS TO THE SKIN AND GIVING IT A ROSY GLOW.

PUMPKIN MASK

Here's another one from the spas that is an excellent moisturizer, skin conditioner, and smoothing body mask. It's rich in vitamin A, plus it contains fruit acid enzymes which work even better than some of the store-bought alpha hydroxies. Pumpkin also has anti-inflammatory properties

Take three cups of fresh pumpkin flesh with seeds and blend for two to three minutes. Stand on some old newspaper and rub the pumpkin mixture into your skin, starting at your feet and working your way up. Let rest for five to ten minutes, then rinse all over. Shower and pat dry.

YEAST AND WHEAT GERM MASK

Mix together a teaspoon of egg, a teaspoon of dried brewer's yeast, one teaspoon of wheat germ, and the contents of one capsule vitamin E. Pat on face and let dry for about fifteen minutes. Rinse with a soft cloth and warm water.

OATMEAL MASKS

You can bet that spas use oatmeal, a lot of it for every skin type. Oatmeal nourishes the skin while providing soothing and calming benefits. They're pricey at spas but mere pennies when done at home. Plus they're easy and quick to prepare.

OILY SKIN

Combine one-half cup of cooked oatmeal with one egg white, one tablespoon of fresh lemon juice, and one-half cup of mashed apple. Mix together into a paste and let set for ten minutes. Wipe off mask with a wet, coarse washcloth.

DRY SKIN

Take a half cup of cooked oatmeal and mix with one teaspoon honey, one egg yolk, and one-half mashed banana. Leave on for fifteen minutes. Then rinse off with cool water.

SENSITIVE SKIN

Combine one-half cup of cooked oatmeal with one whole egg and a teaspoon of almond oil. Leave on face for ten minutes, and then rinse off with tepid water. Pat dry.

GELATIN MASK

Combine one packet of unflavored gelatin or one tablespoon of gelatin with one-half cup of fruit juice (orange, grapefruit, or pineapple). Heat in microwave until warm. Place mixture in the refrigerator and cool until almost set, about thirty minutes. Spread a thin layer of the gel over your face and allow to dry. Peel mask and rinse with cool water.

CHOCOLATE BODY WRAP

Here's a spa treatment that costs $175.00 at a day spa. You can easily do this at home and not even feel guilty while enjoying the rich aroma.

Mix one-quarter cup of honey with three-quarters cup of cocoa powder. Heat the mixture in the microwave until warm but comfortable and apply all over your body. Shower off after twenty minutes.

FRUIT BODY WRAP

As you have probably heard or experienced, there are many natural fruit treatments being used at spas. I love to do the fruit body wrap when I can, not only for the way it makes my skin feel but also for the aroma.

Combine one cup of coconut milk with three cups of crushed pineapple in a blender. Place the mixture in a bowl, then heat in the microwave until warm. Line the bottom of your tub with a blanket, and then put a plastic sheet or shower curtain liner on top of it. Take a seat on the sheet and rub the moisturizing mixture all of your body with your hands or a vegetable brush. Wrap the sheet around you and relax. You will begin to perspire, which is caused by the pineapple. After twenty minutes, remove the plastic and take a shower with cool water. You'll feel wonderful!

PEELS AND POLISHES

ORANGE PEEL

This peel will restore skin tone and even out sunburn. Combine one peeled, chopped orange with two tablespoons of coarse sea salt. Massage mixture on dry skin and let sit for five minutes. Rinse well.

PINEAPPLE BODY POLISH

Special enzymes in pineapples have a wonderful exfoliating effect.

Peel one fresh pineapple and cut into four wedges. While showering, massage wedges into skin, starting at shoulders and working down to feet. Finish by cleansing with a light shower gel, rinsing thoroughly.

ROSE BODY POLISH

Go into the garden and pick a few roses. Combine one-half cup of Epsom salts with scented shower or bath gel to make a paste. Stir in a handful of fresh crushed roses. Rub into damp skin.

SKIN POLISH

Buff skin in the shower with a little brown sugar mixed with some vanilla extract. Rinse and then pat your skin (don't rub) with a thick towel. Use your favorite body lotion mixed with another drop of vanilla extract.

EYE TREATMENTS

Mix a small amount of oatmeal with one-half cup of water and chill in the fridge. Apply to eyes to relieve puffiness.

Take two fennel seed tea bags, run them under warm water, and place them on your eyelids. Fennel is a natural anti-inflammatory.

BEAUTIFUL LASHES

Drizzle a bit of OLIVE OIL on a toothbrush or lash comb and gently comb lashes for a darker, glossy look. Do this at night so it doesn't blur vision or get into your contact lenses.

QUICK TRICKS

- Spread an egg white all over clean skin and let dry. Rinse thoroughly.
- Spread plain yogurt over the face to even out skin tone.
- Remove skin debris with pumpkin filling and nutmeg. Get a can of pumpkin and keep it in the refrigerator. Take a scoop and mix it with about a teaspoon of nutmeg. Follow up with a sugar and honey exfoliant.

- Apply cranberry juice as a cleanser. It's slightly acidic and has antibacterial properties, so it tones while cleansing at the same time.
- Clear up irritated skin with a dollop of whipped cream
- Massage tired muscles with tequila.
- Mash half a ripe peach, and rub it into your face in a circular motion to bring out the glow.
- Crush a peeled tomato, and spread it over your face. Tomatoes contain acids that balance the skin's pH levels and tighten pores.
- Mash half a banana and rub it into clean, dry skin. Leave it on for five minutes. Then rinse well. This mask will leave your skin baby soft, plus the potassium in the bananas will help erase any undereye circles.
- Mash two strawberries and spread them over clean, dry skin. Leave on for five minutes. The strawberries erase blemishes because they're high in salicylic acid, the active ingredient in most over-the-counter acne treatments. The strawberry seeds will slough off rough patches caused by blemishes for instantly smoother skin.

SPA CELLULITE TREATMENTS

There's a very celebrity-popular spa in Mexico that uses this treatment to reduce cellulite. You can do it yourself and save yourself the trip and the bucks.

Crush eight nopal-cactus leaves (available at Latin and natural markets) in a blender. Chill the paste for at least four hours. Rub into the cellulite-ridden areas. Let set for at least ten minutes and then brush off with a vegetable brush or loofah. Rinse.

CELLULITE PASTE

Blend a half cup of coffee beans with a half cup of salt, a tablespoon of kelp, and four tablespoons of olive oil until it becomes a paste.

Apply the mixture over the skin and gently rub in a circular motion with hands or a loofah. Rinse well, and then vigorously pat yourself dry.

Use WARM COFFEE GROUNDS to smooth out cellulite and to exfoliate your skin before using a self-tanner.

SPA WATER TREATMENTS

To energize your body and beat fatigue, use this Swedish water treatment: alternate a minute of warm water with a blast of cool water in the shower.

Get even more invigorated by using some vanilla extract with your cleanser.

Give your face a healthy flush by holding a hot, wet washcloth to your face for a minute. It dilates the blood vessels, creating a hot-flash sensation that brings oxygen right to the skin to revive it.

Sprinkle one cup uncooked oatmeal in your tub to soak away dry, itchy skin.

PREHEAT TOWELS IN THE DRYER WHILE GETTING READY FOR YOUR BATH.

Become friendly with your florist and ask him to save you his **leftover rose petals**. Throw them in your bath for their calming aromatherapy properties.

LEMON TUB SOAK

Mix a tablespoon of lemon juice with one-half cup of baby oil. Add to a warm bath. The lemon will slough off dead skin while the baby oil will leave skin soft and smooth.

MILK BATH TREATMENT

Mix two cups of dry whole-milk powder with one cup of cornstarch. Add one teaspoon of almond or vanilla extract. Stir together in a pretty container, and leave by the tub. Pour in about one-half cup into running bath water to smoothe and soften skin.

After shaving, treat razor burns with an inexpensive **WET TEA BAG**. The cheaper the tea the more tannic acid it has, which will reduce redness.

Treat your bikini line with **OLIVE OIL**. It's full of vitamin E and will help prevent ingrown hairs.

SKIN SOOTHERS

PEACH SMOOTHIE

Peel and mash a ripe peach. Strain to extract all of the juice. Mix juice with an equal amount of heavy whipping cream. Massage into skin and leave on about fifteen minutes. Rinse with warm water.

The gentle fruit acid from the peach and the lactic acid from the cream will soothe and smoothe your skin.

CUCUMBER PARSLEY TONER

This will keep your skin balanced and refreshed. Mix one cup of warm water with two tablespoons of chopped parsley, one-half of a russet potato (scrubbed but not peeled), one-quarter of an unpeeled cucumber, one teaspoon of almond extract, and two teaspoons of lemon juice in a pan. Bring to a boil. Remove from heat, strain, and cool. Apply to skin with a cotton swab.

SUNBURN RELIEVER

Mix one teaspoon of aloe vera gel with one teaspoon of honey. Apply it to the affected area for a few minutes. Then rinse with cool water. This mixture will cool the skin while preventing peeling.

SKIN BUFFER

Blend two cups of crushed macadamia nuts with two sprigs of fresh mint, one-half cup of honey, and one-half teaspoon of almond extract. Mix it all into a paste. Rub all over your body. Rinse and pat skin dry.

ELBOW SOFTENER

Mix one tablespoon of coarse salt with one tablespoon of olive oil. Massage into elbows for one minute, rinse, and then rub half of a fresh cut lemon on the area for thirty seconds. Rinse again.

A MASSAGE THERAPIST SECRET

Mix together four tablespoons of sea salt with one-half cup of olive oil and the juice of one lemon. Massage the mixture over dry skin on the body, not the face. Shower off under warm water with a coarse washcloth.

ANTI-BLOATING TREATMENT

Magnesium chloride found in salt water actually draws out excess water weight. Add one cup of Epsom salts to a warm bath and soak for at least ten to fifteen minutes.

Mix a drop of **MINT EXTRACT** with your lip gloss to get immediate **POUTY LIPS**. Mint stimulates blood flow, making the lips swell temporarily.

STAR SPA TREATMENTS

An employee of the world's most famous spa shared these incredible treatments with me. She says they are the favorites of all the stars.

EGG PACK

Beat an egg until frothy. Apply to a clean, dry face. Let dry on the face, and then rinse thoroughly.

BUTTERMILK AND CORNMEAL EXFOLIANT

Make a paste was one-quarter cup of buttermilk and one-quarter cup of cornmeal. Massage gently over entire face and let set for one minute. Remove with warm water and then apply a warm towel for five minutes.

OREGANO & VANILLA HAIR DETANGLER

One-half cup fresh **OREGANO LEAVES** or two teaspoons **DRIED OREGANO**

One teaspoon **VANILLA EXTRACT**

One cup **WATER**

MICROWAVE above ingredients for thirty to forty seconds.

When cool, STRAIN AND POUR into a spray bottle.

USE after shampooing and conditioning.

LEAVE in refrigerator for up to seven days.

141

Scalp Massage

This is just like a very expensive scalp massage models love!

Soak a towel in a bowl of hot water and five cucumber and five lemon slices. Wring the towel, and wrap it around your head. Relax, and breathe deeply for about ten minutes. Remove towel.

In the palm of your hand, mix a few drops of tea tree oil with a few drops of jojoba oil. Massage your scalp, making circles with your fingers. Shampoo thoroughly.

NATURAL HAIR TREATS

MEDITERRANEAN
HAIR MASK

Massage a teaspoon of olive oil into the scalp for about two to three minutes. Then brush through the hair. Wrap it in a towel for thirty minutes and then shampoo.

SUN STREAKS

Before heading outside, slick your hair into a ponytail lightly coated all over with leave-in conditioner. You'll be amazed at how absolutely sun-kissed your hair looks after thirty minutes of "sun" treatment.

MAKE SOME WAVES

After swimming in the ocean, make a braid or several braids in your hair. When your hair dries, take them out for gorgeous waves.

HAIR SALADS

Mix one tablespoon of apple cider vinegar into a quart of water, and rinse your hair with it when you shower. The vinegar helps to eliminate flaking.

Mix two tablespoons of fresh lemon juice with two tablespoons of apple cider vinegar and one tablespoon of mayonnaise. Slather on dry hair (concentrate on the ends). Leave on for twenty minutes. Rinse with very warm water.

DEEP CLEANSING SHAMPOO

Take the contents of a green tea bag and two tablespoons of olive oil and mix with the juice of a half a lemon and half an orange. Whip in a blender. Then massage into hair and leave on for fifteen minutes. Shampoo and condition.

HAIR REVIVER

Mash a ripe mango with one tablespoon of plain yogurt. Add two egg yolks. Blend and spread all over hair. Cover with plastic wrap or a shower cap and leave on for about twenty minutes. Shampoo thoroughly.

FREEBIE

Can't find a shower cap for your hair treatment? Take a plastic shopping bag, roll up the edges, and pull it into a bunch at the nape or at the top of the head. Secure it with a clip.

SHINE **BOOSTING** CONDITIONER

Brew a cup of tea in a flavor close to your hair color.

Blonde/Chamomile

Brunette/Black currant

Redhead/Orange pekoe

Mix equal parts tea and hair conditioner. Use once or twice a week.

ADD HAIR **VOLUME**

Steep a bag of nettle tea in a cup of water and apply to clean and conditioned hair while damp. Nettle coats and thickens your hair shaft.

DANDRUFF TREATMENT

Boil two tablespoons of dried thyme in a cup of water. Cool, strain, and pour on your scalp. Don't rinse out. Thyme has antiseptic properties.

SPA SOLUTIONS FOR HANDS AND FEET

Mix one-quarter cup of lavender oil with one-half cup of canola oil, and one teaspoon of salt. Massage in to remove dead skin cells. Rinse under tepid water.

Duplicate an expensive foot massage by **STIMULATING PRESSURE POINTS** on your feet by rolling them around on a rubber ball while you bathe.

ATHLETE'S FOOT RELIEF

Mix one tablespoon of baking soda and one-quarter cup of water. Rub between toes to relieve the itch of athlete's foot. Leave mixture on until it dries. Rinse and dry feet completely.

NEAT NAILS

Mix together one cup of milk or cream with one tablespoon of moisturizer. Warm and microwave. When warm but comfortable to the touch, soak hands for fifteen minutes.

Rub jojoba oil or almond oil on your cuticles and fingers to keep them healthy and to keep nails from splitting.

Get your nails white by dipping them in half a lemon for a minute or two. The citric acid naturally bleaches tips.

THE **POWERFUL** PINEAPPLE

It's a great fruit with citric qualities that many spas use.

Pineapple Cuticle Treatment

Use this treatment before pushing back your cuticles.

¼ cup pineapple
½ teaspoon apple cider vinegar
one teaspoon vegetable oil
one tablespoon honey
one egg yolk

Mix together and apply to hands, concentrating on cuticles. Wrap hands in plastic gloves or plastic wrap. Leave on for fifteen minutes. Remove plastic and rinse with warm water.

PINEAPPLE
FOOT SMOOTHER

Use once or twice a week to keep your feet sandal-ready!

One-half cup chopped **PINEAPPLE**
One-half **APPLE** (unpeeled)
One-half **LEMON** (peeled)
One-quarter **GRAPEFRUIT** (peeled)
two teaspoons **ANISE EXTRACT**
one teaspoon **SALT**

Mix ingredients together. Rub mixture on feet, concentrating on heels. Wrap feet in plastic and leave on for twenty to thirty minutes. Rinse with warm water.

ALWAYS BE CAREFUL WHEN APPLYING ANY ESSENTIAL OIL TO SKIN, ESPECIALLY SENSITIVE SKIN. **TEST IT FIRST.**

HAND AND ARM THERAPY

There's a wonderful (but expensive) Tahitian scrub that you can make yourself for under a dollar.

Grind one-half cup shelled walnuts into a powder. Add two tablespoons of olive oil and one tablespoon of honey. Rub over hands and lower arms for a few minutes. Rinse well.

SPA PEDICURE

Toss five bags of green tea into a basin of hot water. Let cool until comfortable and put both feet and ankles in. Let soak until water cools completely. Rub fresh mint leaves over your toes and feet. Apply olive oil to seal in moisture.

ESSENTIAL OILS

Here are some essential oils that spas use and you should collect.

Lavender

Helps with burns, sprains, healing wounds, and calming the mind and body. Use it on your pillow, or dab it around your room when you want to relax. Add a couple of drops to your bath.

Eucalyptus

Aids in clearing up skin infections and is a natural insect repellent. Put some inside your pillow to help you breathe more easily, especially if you have a cold. Add a couple of leaves to boiling water to steam your face.

Tea Tree Oil

Helps cold sores, oily skin, athlete's foot, and blemishes. Use it straight from the bottle.

Geranium

Helps fade broken capillaries. Use it at night to heal bruises.

Grapefruit

Tones skin and tissues and helps with bloating. You'll love it as a bath oil. Use about ten drops under running water.

Peppermint

Soothes digestion and is cool and refreshing. Apply it in the air or on the skin.

Chapter 15

MODEL SAVINGS

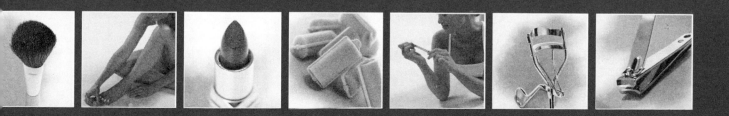

SECRETS FROM BEHIND THE RUNWAYS

Most everyone assumes that for a model to look great, it has to have cost a lot, taken a lot of time, or it's just that she's been naturally blessed. Let me set you straight from behind the runway. Models are apt to do things quicker, cheaper, and more efficiently because they've learned how from the experts. Here are great tips from the modeling world that will help even if you're not planning to strut the catwalk in the near future.

IT'S THE ART OF ILLUSION

Models use henna and temporary tattoos to achieve a look. It's an inexpensive way to see if you really like it.

Temporary tattoos are used widely, because, quite simply, most modeling agencies don't allow tattoos. The models who have them usually have to cover them up with heavy concealer.

You can find temporary tattoos at lots of stores, including drugstores and costume and novelty shops. They're fun, painless, and totally removable.

There are also salons that will do a henna tattoo. They last longer (two to four weeks) and they have been around forever.

MODEL TRICKS

Cindy Crawford keeps her skin fresh and moist by making a spritzer using equal amounts of milk and bottled water. She puts it into a spray bottle and shakes it up. Cindy says she uses it all day, especially after workouts. After spraying, she just wipes the excess off with a tissue.

Tyra Banks is honest in admitting to having a bad habit of nail-biting. She does what many models before her have done to cure themselves of this habit. She dips her fingers in vinegar or Tabasco sauce. It definitely has kept her fingers out of her mouth.

James King's favorite lip moisturizer is honey, which she applies over her lipstick for extra shine. Then she gently blots it so that it looks like it's part of her lipstick.

MODEL MAKEUP TOOLS

FINGERS

The best makeup tool is located right at the end of your hand. Forego those fancy applicators and start finger-painting. That's what the top makeup artists do.

For a sexy smudge on your eyes, use your pinky and soften the line.

For a brightening effect on the eye, pat on color on the inner corner of the eyes to the upper, outer quadrant. Always pat, never rub or pull at the eye area.

SPOONS

Carefully hold a clean spoon against the upper eyelid with the hollow side turned in and the bottom edge lined up with the base of your lashes. Apply mascara using short, quick strokes. Extra product will end up on the spoon, not clumped on your lashes.

Are you a klutz when it comes to using a lash curler? No problem. You can get a great curl by heating a metal spoon briefly with the hairdryer and then applying the outside of the spoon to your upper lashes. Hold for about ten seconds, and your lashes are instantly and perfectly curled!

HOW MODELS DISGUISE IMPERFECTIONS

Prepare the area with a drop of moisturizer mixed with a drop or two of eye-redness reliever. This will allow the concealer to properly stick to the skin. Next, take a very small brush and dip into concealer. Gently brush over the blemish. Apply foundation. Then reapply concealer. Gently pat over with loose powder to keep the blemish covered.

TRICKS OF THE TRADE

PERFECT (LOOKING) SKIN

To create the look of flawless skin, wrap a pressed powder puff around your pointer finger. Dip it into loose powder and carefully roll it onto your skin.

HIGH CHEEKBONES

Models get the illusion of high cheekbones by applying foundation one shade deeper than their regular foundation shade. They apply it just under the cheekbone.

BIGGER EYES

Use a pale, shimmery eye shadow in a peach or pink shade on the lid and in the inner corner of the eye, right near the bridge of the nose. It creates a brightening effect. It's perfect by itself, or over another eye shadow color.

HERE'S **THE MODEL'S WAY** TO CURL YOUR LASHES. CLAMP YOUR CURLER AT THE BASE OF YOUR LASHES AND THEN **"WALK"** IT OUT TO THE TIP. BE SURE TO CLAMP DOWN ALONG THE WAY.

Always soften your liner after applying it with a cotton swab. Pat over the line to achieve the smoky effect

Seal your eyeliner with powdered shadow in a closely matching shade

BRIGHT TEETH

Make your teeth look whiter by using a bright shade of lipstick. The color contrast will make your teeth look like you've had a whitening treatment.

LUSCIOUS LIPS

Open a vitamin E capsule with a pin and squeeze the contents on your fingertip. Use it as a gloss and to treat chapped lips. Wipe off the flakes with a toothbrush.

Coat lips with foundation and let it dry. Apply lip gloss and blot.

POUTY LIPS

Want to save big money on collagen injections? Here's how the models give the illusion of pouty lips.

- Add shine over your lipstick. Shine makes anything look bigger. Run it along your lips with your pointer finger because it's the most precise finger. Start at the center, which is the fullest part of your mouth, and then smooth out towards the corners.
- Warm some bag balm in the microwave and gently pat on your lip after it's warm but comfortable to the touch. Using a baby's toothbrush, gently brush your lip in a circular motion. This will not only take away the chapping but it also will swell the lips temporarily, making your lips look fuller.

MORE LIP TRICKS

- Always wipe off lip balm before applying lipstick. Lips must be clean, or the lipstick will go on unevenly.
- Never apply a hard lip pencil to lips. Soften the tip by warming it up for a few seconds between your fingers.
- Make lips look smaller by applying concealer on lip rim. Draw an outline that's just inside the natural lip line.
- Keep lipstick off teeth by inserting a tissue into your mouth with your finger and then drawing out excess lipstick.
- Darken your lip gloss by putting a little bit of dark brown shadow before application.
- Conceal a lipstick's lightness by applying a neutral lipliner all over the lip.
- Update lipstick with a cool blue base. Create it with a little bit of blue eye shadow. Mix a little

into your lipstick until you've created the right shade.

- Models are told to sip through a straw to protect their teeth from stain-makers like coffee, cola, tea, and red wine.
- At photo shoots, lipsticks are often kept on top of a cool soda bottle. It keeps them from turning to mush. Makeup artists are known to pack their makeup in small zippered plastic bags kept in chilled gel packs.

NATURAL LOOKING LIPS

When models need to look like they have no makeup on (i.e.,that "natural" look) here's what they do: apply lip balm and then apply neutral pencil over it.

PETROLEUM JELLY GIVES LIPS A NATURAL GLOSS.

MODEL EYES

Hold your mascara wand in a vertical position while applying mascara. It will give your lashes more volume. This method also replaces liner because it creates a natural line.

Wake up your eyes by applying eyeliner thinly at the inner eye and thicker at the outer eye.

SHADOW **TRICK**

Have your eye shadow perform double duty. Apply it wet to get a smoky look. Don't use water because it will crack once it's dry. Apply a drop of eye redness reliever to your brush, and then dip into the shadow. This is done at photo shoots because the eye redness reliever turns the powder into a paste. It looks perfect and, even better, it lasts.

SAVING FACE

Wake up your complexion with an ice cube. Rub it over your face and watch the circulation increase. That's a glow, girl.

Blend lipstick into cheeks for a **NATURAL GLOW**. Use your finger so that the heat of your body temperature will help blend in the color. Never go beyond the outer corner of the eyes.

GET THE PERFECT BLUSH COLOR

Match your blush to the skin inside your lower lip.

MODEL HAIR TRICKS

QUICK TRICKS FOR **FAT HAIR**

Simply switch your part to the opposite side. It gives hair an instant lift.

Comb styling gel through slightly damp hair. Twist sections around your finger and hold them with clips. Blow dry on the lowest setting. Remove the clips, and lift your hair at the roots.

Turn your head upside down and blow dry hair while fluffing. Flip over and smooth the cuticle.

SHINY HAIR

Spray anti-frizz/shine serum on a large fluffy makeup brush. Use the largest brush you can find, and make sure it's used only for hair. Brush it all over hair for a mirror-like finish.

Rub a bit of hair conditioner in your hands and gently pat all over your head.

AVOID LEAVING A **DENT IN YOUR HAIR** BY SLIPPING A TISSUE UNDER YOUR HAIR CLIPS WHILE APPLYING MAKEUP.

STRAIGHT HAIR

Here's how to get hair perfectly straight without a flat iron. Clip hair against one side of your head and blow dry. Repeat on the other side of your head.

FREEBIE
Keep a comb between your flat iron and your scalp so you don't burn yourself.

When **STRAIGHTENING HAIR** with a blow dryer, start at the ends and work your way up. Always point the dryer down on top of the hair to seal in the cuticle and make the hair flatter.

MODEL BODY TRICKS

MODEL LEGS

- Keep weight on one leg, and bring your other leg forward so one foot is crossed in front of the other, then bend you knee slightly to create a slim line.
- Wear sheer dark hose. Light colors make legs look heavier.
- Don't cross your legs. It hurts circulation and causes spider veins.
- Massage your legs with lotion every night in a circular motion.
- Use creams containing cocoa butter.
- Sleep in cotton leggings after applying a thick layer of lotion. In the morning, your legs will be super smooth.

Models prevent **RAZOR RASH** by loosening hairs before shaving. Scrubbing with a loofah or coarse washcloth also takes away the top layer of skin to allow a smooth surface for shaving.

Dark Skin Patches

Apply a lemon half to knees and heels where skin is thicker and darker. The citric acid bleaches and softens. Let it set for ten to fifteen minutes. Rinse off with a wet washcloth.

Soft Skin

Models get extra-soft legs for those extremely close shots by applying a facemask on their legs. Use it once a week all over your legs. Let it set for ten minutes and then rinse off in the shower.

Firm Legs

Here's what models do before a swimsuit shoot to make their legs look sleek and slim. Apply dried seaweed sheets to wet legs. It's available at health food stores and natural supermarkets. Apply a blow dryer until the seaweed dries. Then peel off seaweed.

Cellulite Remover

Models apply warm coffee grounds (make sure it contains caffeine). They massage it in with a vegetable brush in a circular motion; let it set for five minutes, and then rinse off.

Model's Trick for Stranding in High Heels

Tape your second toe (the one next to your big toe) on top of your third toe to help high heels feel more comfortable. This trick takes some pressure off the feet.

Ingrown Hairs

See those little bumps on your knees and bikini line? They're actually ingrown hairs. Get rid of them by scrubbing the area with a mesh shower puff. Use a circular motion.

PHOTO FINISH SHAVE

- TO SHAVE LIKE THE MODELS DO, **SHAVE IN THE MORNING** WHEN LEGS ARE LESS PUFFY.

- LET LEGS ABSORB WATER FOR A COUPLE OF MINUTES TO **OPEN UP THE FOLLICLES**.

- USE **HAIR CONDITIONER** FOR A SMOOTHER SHAVE.

- RINSE LEGS IN **COLD WATER** TO CLOSE THE PORES.

Photo Shoot Trick

Apply hair shine serum to your legs. Mix hair serum with a little bronzing powder, concentrating on shins and the tops of the thighs. This highlights the bones and creates definition.

MODEL ARMS

Models use face-firming masks to tighten their arms. Simply apply the mask to the backs of your arms and let it dry. Then rinse off.

Models get rid of bumps on the back of their arms by using AHA creams. The success lies in the cream's ability to gently slough off the dead cell layers.

TO HEAL BRUISES QUICKLY, BREAK OPEN A VITAMIN K CAPSULE AND TAP THE CONTENTS INTO THE BRUISE.

MODEL EATING

Trust me, model eating is not just diet soda and bubble gum. There are lots of tricks that models use.

What does **Gisele** eat for that "oh my goodness, how did she get that body" look? This is what all the models from Brazil that I've worked with do.

Breakfast: Fruit, grain bread, coffee.
Lunch: Salad, fish or meat, quinoa, and dessert. It's their largest meal of the day.
Dinner: Stew, salad, bread, and cheese.

Heidi Klum drinks soy shakes and runs wind sprints before each Victoria's Secret shoot and runway show.

MUSTS FOR MODELS BEFORE A PHOTO SHOOT

• Never skip breakfast.
• Don't go more than four hours without eating.
• Fill half of plate with vegetables.

161

The Day Before

- Drink as much water as possible to detox your body.
- Add an extra workout of no less than thirty minutes.

MODEL EMERGENCIES

OVERPLUCKING

Sometimes makeup artists go overboard and pluck, pluck, pluck away. It can get so bad that the models can't remember what their natural brows originally looked like.

When this happens to you, try the following:

- Leave your brows alone for three weeks to see if the hairs will grow back.
- Comb brows up and out. Snip off any extra long hairs.
- Don't go outside the brow line, but use a soft pencil to fill in very sparse spots.

- Shadow over the brow in a closely matched shade so the brow won't look so harsh.

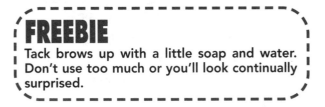

FREEBIE
Tack brows up with a little soap and water. Don't use too much or you'll look continually surprised.

NO BRA, NO PROBLEM

Models carry tape for such occasions. One or two strips of electrical tape are carried from one armpit to the other. Just follow where the bottom of your bra would go. Destick the tape on some fabric or plain white paper so that it doesn't hurt when it's pulled off.

NOSE BUMPS

Lots of models have slight bumps that can easily be disguised. After applying foundation, dip a brush into eye shadow that's slightly darker than your skin tone. On each side of your nose, draw a light line along the sides, stopping at the bridge.

BREAKOUT PREVENTION

Models who tend to break out and know they have a modeling assignment the next day eat one or two antacid tablets before going to bed. They balance the acid in the skin and help to stop breakouts.

BREAKOUT **RASH**

Apply sliced cucumbers to the rash. It has anti-inflammatory properties to tone down redness. Apply tea tree oil as a toner.

SHAVING **EMERGENCY**

Put pressure on the cut for five minutes with a tissue soaked in a nasal decongestant spray like Afrin, which stops blood flow by constricting blood vessels.

RUNWAY HAIR

Models, who are going for that "at the beach" look take a clear, carbonated soda like Sprite and pour it into a spray bottle. Then they lightly spray it on the ends of curly or wavy hair.

To make hair immediately shiny and get residue out, make a paste from baking soda and water. Apply it to hair for twenty minutes. Rinse out thoroughly. This is especially good for getting rid of chlorine. Models use it after photo shoots that involve posing in chlorinated swimming pools.

Make your style last a little longer by keeping fingers, brushes, and styling products out of your hair for less buildup.

Refresh your style with a blow dryer set on cool.

Bring hair **BACK TO LIFE** by rolling it in opposite directions.

RUNWAY LEGS

To make models legs look instantly tan, we rub a dry oil mixed with bronzing powder all over the legs.

If there's more time, a self-tanner is used, mixed with a small amount of moisturizer to ensure an even appearance.

THIN **LIPS**

A small amount of gloss or pearlized eye shadow in the center of the bottom lip will make the lips appear fuller and pouty.

> Dab light EYE SHADOW or HIGHLIGHTING CREAM right above the bow of the lip and blend slightly.

TIRED EYES

When a model's eyes become bloodshot, a cotton ball saturated with eye drops that are kept in the refrigerator is gently placed on the eye. It cools the eyes and makes the redness disappear in less than a minute.

REFRESHING MAKEUP

Use this model technique to refresh your eye makeup without having to reapply it all. Use a cotton swab and non-oily makeup remover to take off any makeup that has smudged under your eyes. Then lightly pat on an alcohol-free toner and concealer.

BIGGER LASHES

Bend your mascara wand at a 90-degree angle. You'll get more control and will be able to push the wand through each of your lashes instead of from the side.

UNMENTIONABLE **ACNE**

Toothpaste mixed with cocoa butter is used by models to prevent butt pimples.

MODELS USE BODY OIL SPRAY ON THEIR CLEAVAGE. IT MAKES THE **SKIN LOOKS SEXY AND GLOSSY**. YOU CAN DO THE SAME FOR YOUR OWN TREASURE CHEST.

BELIEVABLE BRONZER

How do those models look so naturally tan? It's called the fine art of bronzing.

Here are the rules:

- Bronzer should never be more than two shades darker than the skin's natural color.
- Creams work best for dry skin while powder is a better choice for oily or combination skin.
- Liquid formulas are never advised.
- A blush brush makes it easier to control coverage.

To apply cream bronzers, fingers are really the best applicators. It helps the bronzer blend into the skin. Only use bronzer on bones, not the entire face. Focus on highlighting the cheekbones, bones above the temples, and the bridge of the nose, mimicking a natural tan.

To minimize contrast, run the bronzer down the center of the neck into the cleavage.

Drugstores have excellent bronzers. It's never necessary to spend a lot on bronzer since the intent is for shading over pigment.

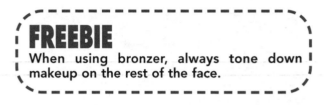

FREEBIE

When using bronzer, always tone down makeup on the rest of the face.

Chapter 16

CELEBRITY SAVINGS

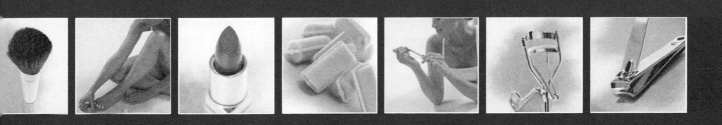

SURE THEY LOOK PERFECT

How do those celebrities look so gorgeous? Of course, they have lots of time and money to keep up their looks, but they also have secret beauty tricks that surprisingly don't cost very much. They pick up the tricks of the trade while they're backstage and behind those runways. They don't always talk about these tricks because some of them are less than elegant— things like hemorrhoid cream and sliced potatoes are not good for the image or conducive to endorsements.

Although you may never see them using these products, you better believe if it works, they will use anything and everything. And the results are well worth it. You won't see their dark roots, their puffy eyes, their bloated tummies. Celebrities occasionally are willing to share the tips on how they like to save. It makes them feel like they're putting one over on the beauty industry. Plus, if they've been happy with a drug-store product that works well on them, they're loathe to change. They've got their favorites and here are some of them.

BEAUTY TRICKS

Ashley Judd keeps her lips puckery perfect by rubbing a pineapple chunk on them followed by a dab of petroleum jelly. The fruit acids slough off dead skin and the petroleum jelly seals in the moisture.

Britney Spears treats her blemishes by steaming them with lemon herbal tea and boiling water. She boils a big pot and puts her face over it until it cools. It also clears clogged pores.

Drew Barrymore's favorite beauty tool is a eyelash curler. Her lashes grow down, so she really "opens her eyes" with her curler. Drew likes to heat the curler briefly with her blow dryer so that the curl stays in.

Alyssa Milano's trademark is her perfectly shaped eyebrows. To achieve them, she matches up her eye's iris and tapers them down to the corner of her outer eye.

Sarah Michelle Gellar emphasizes her eyes and lips with just the right amount of blush. She gets the right contour by following the lines of her cheekbones with her blush brush.

Gwyneth Paltrow plays up her eyes with sparkly gray eye shadow and a soft kohl gray pencil. She rims it around both her upper and lower lashes.

Jennifer Lopez uses shimmering creams and powders all over her body and face. Her lips are always highly glossed.

Courteney Cox Arquette keeps her skin looking flawless and oil-free with rice-paper powdered tissues. They can be found at drugstores or beauty supply shops.

Angie Harmon opens up her deep-set eyes with a well-groomed brow. It creates a lift and brings the eye forward. She chooses a light shadow and defined lash line.

Christina Aguilera widens her eyes by only applying shadow on the outer corners and lightening her eyelids with gloss.

Mariah Carey mixes a drop of mint extract with a dab of lip gloss before applying. The mint stimulates blood flow and enhances lip color. Make sure you have no sensitivity to mint.

Lisa Kudrow soaks thick and smooth paper napkins in almond oil and keeps them in plastic bags when she travels. They moisturize and refresh her skin and leave a heavenly fragrance.

Singer and actress **Brandy** uses an antibiotic ointment (like Neosporin) overnight when she has an acne rash.

Naomi Campbell accents her lips with Jell-O. It's a great stain. Dip a moistened cotton swab into Jell-O powder in the color of your choice. Leave it on for about three to four minutes and then lick it off. Sometimes she tops it of with gloss.

One of **TYRA BANKS**' favorite exercises is running. Afterwards she treats her feet to this soothing foot soak.

Fill a basin with warm water and add one-quarter cup of granulated sugar, two tablespoons of almond oil, and three drops of rosemary oil. She then massages her feet with her fingers. After ten minutes of rubbing, she pats her feet dry and puts on socks to seal in the softness.

Rene Russo minimizes her high forehead with this foundation trick that you can copy. Brush a foundation that is a shade darker than your regular shade along the hairline from the tops of the ears to the center of the forehead. Blend so that the color disappears into the hairline.

Natalie Portman is not one to waste her money on a lot of stuff. She says that she can do without the materialism that goes along with her industry, and feels that her money can go to better places. But that doesn't mean that she doesn't love style. She gets big compliments on the many earrings that she buys at Target.

Melanie Griffith loves natural beauty treatments, but as a mom she can't just pick up and go at a moment's notice. That's why she loves to do some of these treatments in her own bathroom. Her skin-smoothing favorite is to mash an avocado with a few drops of witch hazel and apply it to her face in a circular motion. She leaves it on for about twenty minutes while she relaxes in her bath. Then she rinses with warm water. It leaves her skin feeling silky.

Helen Hunt uses this trick to make her eyes prominent. She brushes her brow hairs straight up and then sets them with hair spray. She then traces a thin line of taupe eye shadow along the upper edge of her brow. This lifts the eye and makes it appear larger.

Jewel uses shimmery lip gloss on her eye lids.

CELEBRITY WORKOUTS

Gwyneth Paltrow stays slim with yoga. It can be done anywhere, and gives her that lovely, graceful gait.

Mariah Carey claims her dancing is strenuous exercise, and she gets a great workout on stage.

Beyonce Knowles dances for thirty to forty-five minutes each day and does an amazing five

Reese Witherspoon relies on this tennis ball trick to relax her muscles after a strenuous workout. You can replicate it at home and use it to relax after a day of sitting at a desk.

- Tape two tennis balls together with strong tape and lie on a mat or carpet.

- Place the balls under your back. Roll your body up and down, keeping the balls on either side of the spine. This roll will give you a wonderful massage and take out any knots.

hundred sit ups. She boosts her energy with lots of water. Since she loves to show her great legs on stage, she does twenty leg lunges, holding five pound weights.

Scrubs star **Sarah Chalke** prefers hiking to the gym. She claims it's the only calm way to work out, much more so than a crowded gym with loud music. Plus, it really strengthens her lower body.

Catherine Bell doesn't have time to go to the gym, so she tries to get in out about ten minutes of exercise during studio breaks shooting hoops. She works up a good sweat and feels energized.

Renee Zellweger stretches and lunges to trim her abs and butt. She has literally sculpted her body. She chooses clothing to accentuate her hard work. A pencil skirt gives her a trim lower body and defines her small waist.

FREEBIE

How did she lose all that weight?

Everyone knows that RENEE ZELLWEGER packed on about twenty pounds to star in *Bridget Jones' Diary.* **She flushed it away by drinking lots of water and following a basic high-protein diet. She ate a fruit salad for breakfast, a green salad for lunch, and then grilled fish for dinner.**

Rebecca Romijn-Stamos rates her favorite exercise as swimming, especially the freestyle stroke.

Sarah Jessica Parker bikes in Central Park and maintains her weight by having five to seven mini meals each day. Since she lives in New York, she walks everywhere. To get the most out her walking, Sarah Jessica squeezes her buttocks in each and every step. She believes a gym is not necessary when you're able to get outdoors.

Christina Applegate spins and keeps her energy up with orange juice.

Jennifer Love Hewitt loves kickboxing because it uses all her muscles and gives her energy.

Julia Roberts' one big meal of the day is always breakfast. She exercises by losing herself in dancing and jogging. Julia's favorite food? A big baked potato with fat-free cottage cheese, fresh herbs, and Butter Buds.

Jamie-Lynn Sigler of *The Sopranos* works her hips and thighs out with lunges. She does them when she brushes her teeth, when she's memorizing her lines, and even at crossing lights. Try to do ten on each leg, three times a day. She has overcome anorexia and now believes in maintaining a normal weight.

Model/actress **Rebecca Romijn-Stamos** hates doing ab work so much that she does two hundred crunches at a time, three times a week.

Lie on your back with your hands behind your head. Lift your shoulders and extend your left leg as you bring your right knee in to your chest, touching it with your left elbow. Hold to the count of three. Switch sides and do the same. Do no more than five to ten reps each, especially if you're just starting out.

Angel star **Charisma Carpenter** loves healthy foods, especially cottage cheese. She tones her body by playing lots of tennis.

Janet Jackson's problem was loving to eat, and especially loving to eat out. She even admits to having battled with bulimia and anorexia. She dramatically changed her appearance by switching to a vegetarian-based diet and started running, doing sit-ups, and boxing.

TOMATO PORE MINIMIZER

Leeza Gibbons said she prefers homemade beauty remedies to spa getaways so that she can have more time with her kids.

Her favorite recipe is to take a tomato and cut it into thick slices. She allows the juice and seeds to drain and then mashes the pulp with a fork. She applies it to her face, covers it with a warm washcloth, and then sits for fifteen minutes before washing with warm water.

Jenna Elfman credits her body to taking ballet lessons three times a week, drinking ten glasses of water a day, avoiding sugar, and getting nine hours of sleep a night.

Model/actress Lauren Hutton claims that she's not that disciplined when it comes to exercise. She does a few stretches at home for no more than ten to fifteen minutes and then she walks everywhere at a brisk pace.

CELEBRITY HAIR SECRETS

Have you ever wondered how Melanie Griffith has maintained such great hair after so many dos and colors? She relies on almond oil. She just puts a few drops on her fingers and scrunches it into her hair, leaves it on for twenty minutes, and then shampoos and conditions.

When Julia Roberts decides to go curly, she scrunches her hair with a curl-enhancing gel just after shampooing, and curls with a curling iron in a vertical direction.

Lucy Liu's great waves are the result of a blunt cut with slight layering at the ends for movement. Her hair is blown dry, using a round brush and pinned in larger pin curls. When the pins come out, her hair is gently finger-styled.

Drew Barrymore's secret hair trick for less-than-perfect hair days is to part her hair in the middle, pull one side back, and then secure it with a big sparkling barrette. You can find great ones at flea markets, or use a big pin. Attach it to your hair with bobby pins.

Ananda Lewis' beautiful long hair is a combination of using Herbal Essences conditioning balm and this great secret: when she's having a bad hair day, she applies olive oil over the top of her hair to calm it down and give it shine.

Here's what makes up **MICHELLE PFEIFFER**'s beauty treatments for her hair.

Two **egg yolks**

One-quarter cup **honey**

One ounce **rum**

One ounce **apple cider vinegar**
added to 7 ounces **water**

She warms the honey, lets it cool, and applies it to her roots. Then she mixes the egg yolks and rum, and smothers her hair shaft with the mixture. She covers her head with a shower cap for twenty minutes. Michelle then rinses with water, shampoos as usual, and rinses with the vinegar and water combination.

Britney Spears' split ends get treated with castor oil. She rubs it between her palms and applies it to the ends.

James King puts her own highlights in her hair. Here's how: she cuts out the top of an old straw hat, pulls her hair through the hole, then pours cooled chamomile tea on her hair and sits out in the sun for about thirty minutes. She then washes and conditions.

Mandy Moore adds shine to her hair with a whole egg and one-half cup of honey. She puts the mixture on dry hair, combs it through, and leaves it on for about an hour. Then she washes it out. It keeps her hair shiny and soft.

Moore also had a lot of bad hair days growing up. She was the victim of too many permanents. Here's the conditioning trick that fixed her damaged hair: pour jojoba oil all over dry hair, concentrating on the ends. Leave it on about ten minutes, and then rinse it through with very warm water. Shampoo and condition lightly.

Reese Witherspoon's hair tends to "puff" up. She uses baby oil to make it behave.

Molly Sims rates avocado as her favorite conditioner. She mashes a ripe avocado in a bowl and then applies it to unwashed hair. Molly leaves it on for twenty minutes before shampooing thoroughly.

Melissa Joan Hart loves the smell of lavender. Every day she applies lavender oil (available at health food stores and natural supermarkets) to her hair, concentrating on her ends to tame and scent.

Jennifer Aniston uses Mane 'n Tail shampoo once a week. This shampoo was originally marketed to silken show horses' manes.

Tori Spelling loves to mix a tablespoon of lemon juice with a tablespoon of peroxide and apply it to damp hair. Then she sits out in the sun for twenty minutes to lighten it.

Deborah Messing lets her just-curled hair cool before finger-combing; she finishes with a silicone spray for shine.

Carmen Electra mashes a ripe avocado, puts it in her hair, and then sits out in the sun for a half hour. After rinsing, she's left with soft and shiny hair.

CELEBRITY SOLUTIONS

Think you're the only one with bad skin, kinky hair, or something worse? Everyone has them, even the most super of models and the sought-after celebrity.

Tara Reid minimizes large pores and gets rid of blackheads by using vitamin A powder mixed with her cleanser. It helps prevent her pores from getting clogged.

Pro-surfing champ and model **Malia Jones** fixes the damage that the sun and the ocean inflict on her hair by using hot oil treatments every week. To moisturize her body, Malia uses baby oil, perfect after a long day at the beach.

Model **Gisele Bundchen** never uses soap, only makeup remover and water to keep her skin from losing moisture.

Cameron Diaz started modeling with no style, feathered hair, and a comb in her back pocket. Now she's a role model. She adds funky touches like a big flower to her elegant shoes. She keeps slim with lots of hot salsa and water.

BLOCKBUSTER FIGURES

Penelope Cruz uses diet Popsicles to fool her sweet tooth. It numbs her tongue and gets rid of that nasty coating. Her favorite flavor is lime. At only ten calories, she lets herself have a treat up to ten times a day.

Jessica Alba comes from a family that is heavily overweight. She actually started cooking for herself at age twelve so she would not have the same problems. Her breakfast is usually an egg white omelet and fruit or cottage cheese with a peach. For lunch she chooses a salad. For dinner she has vegetables and chicken or fish. During the day, she picks dried fruit or frozen yogurt.

Whitney Houston gets gorgeous shimmer on her arms and legs by making a lotion out of a tablespoon of baby oil mixed with two tablespoon of bronzing powder.

Lisa Marie, former model and actress (*Planet of the Apes*), only eats foods that give her energy and help her feel good. When she began eating this way, she stopped having to diet. She claims that when she eats healthfully—eating clean proteins and vegetables—she feels balanced, and her nervous system is calm. She eats a lot of organic vegetables, fruits, homemade food, salmon, and salads.

Sandra Bullock's secret to staying slim is to eat slowly. She usually finishes her meal ten minutes after her friends.

When **Jennifer Lopez** gets ready for a role, she relies on chicken and fish salads.

Jennifer Love Hewitt's always struggled with sweets, especially her mom's cupcakes. Now when her sweet tooth strikes, she grabs a piece of fruit.

Halle Berry doesn't maintain her body with her number one downfall, the love of potato chips. But she's not one to deny herself, so sensible Halle eats her chips baked. And she's trained her taste buds to enjoy low-fat pretzels.

Even celebrities get sick of constant dieting and watching their weight. Look at **JENNIFER LOPEZ**. Her weight tends to yo-yo, and yet she wears her clothes proudly no matter if it's up or down. The same goes for **KATE WINSLET** and **ALICIA SILVERSTONE**, and it means that they're real people just like us.

STAR SECRETS
FOR THE RIGHT LOOK

SKIRTS cut on the bias in a light fabric (like a knit) give a **SLIM LOOK**.

Long **NARROW** skirts with a drop waist disguise a **BULGE**.

A **TAILORED JACKET** with just enough padding makes your shoulders look **WIDER** than your **HIPS**.

Wear pants that skim the body and fall just a bit long, and, of course, **DARKER IS ALWAYS MORE SLIMMING**.

Chapter 17

SHOPPING BARGAINS

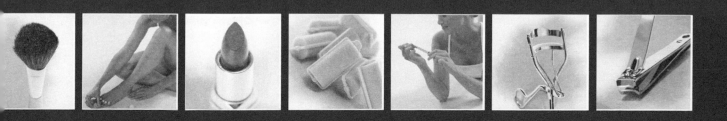

PLAYING THE SHOPPING GAME

It is a game if you're a bargain hunter like me. It's relaxing, it's competitive, and you seem to enjoy it more when you've snagged it at a bargain price.

Don't let them get you! The stores will do anything and everything to get you to buy. Here's their game.

They will play relaxing music.

There will be scents that will make you want to stay, relax, and buy.

The colors will make you pay more. Pink is the #1 favorite of packaging experts.

The item you're most likely to pick will be at your eye level or lower.

It will be priced right. Nine is the most popular final digit. It makes the buyer think she's getting a good deal.

It's touchable. Buyers like to feel fabrics before buying.

There will be a coupon to cinch the deal.

DISCOUNT BAGS IN LEATHER ARE HARD TO FIND. YOU CAN DO BETTER WITH CANVAS OR FABRIC. MICROFIBER IS LIGHTWEIGHT AND DURABLE. PLUS, ITS PRICE RANGE IS NOT EVIDENT IN ITS APPEARANCE.

SHOPPING MISSES

POORLY PLACED **BUTTONS**

When fasteners on a shirt or sweater are too widely spaced above and below the breast area, it will gap unattractively.

EXCESS FABRIC

It kills the look and fit. In the industry it's called a "grin" when excess fabric hits the crotch. It's not a happy look.

BAD **LINING**

Look for cheap fabric lining (like rayon). It can shrink once it's dry cleaned and ruin the look of the garment. The wrong lining can make a garment look matronly.

UNFLATTERING **POCKETS**

When pockets are too small, they can actually make your butt look bigger. When they're stitched on too high, they flatten out your butt.

HERE'S WHAT YOU NEED TO DO TO TAKE CHARGE

Shop with a list. You need certain things. A list will keep you from getting sidetracked.

Compare prices. Try to get the best deal, but don't buy something just because it's on sale. If you have to talk yourself into something, then you won't wear it enough.

Use a three-way mirror. You want to look great at every angle for anything you wear to be truly worth buying.

Don't let salespeople make you buy anything. You know what looks good on you.

Find things that are easy to care for. Check the labels for instructions. If something is a good buy, but constantly has to be sent to the cleaners, it's a budget-breaker.

Don't buy anything that pulls, bunches, rides up, or makes noise when you walk. You should be able to pull an inch of fabric to allow you to eat, move, and be comfortable.

THE LESS LEATHER

ON AN INEXPENSIVE SHOE, THE MORE EXPENSIVE IT WILL LOOK.

THE BEST TIME TO HIT

A SALE IS FRIDAY NIGHT. STORES ARE USUALLY NOT CROWDED AND VERY OFTEN ARE OPEN LATER WHEN THERE'S A SALE.

TAKE ADVANTAGE OF

PRESEASON SALES. THE PRICE MAY NOT COME DOWN IN SEASON. THIS IS ESPECIALLY TRUE OF SWIMSUITS, CASHMERE, AND OUTERWEAR.

DRUGSTORES

You can save big money and avoid being hassled or ignored by shopping drugstores for your beauty supplies. The cosmetics at the cosmetic counter are often made with the same technology as the drugstore brands. Some are even made in the same factories, and owned by the same parent companies. The only differences are packaging, marketing, advertising, sales help, counter leasing, and, of course, price.

But how do you find the right shade without opening any bottles? Here's how you do it.
Check the label.
You'll see brief descriptions that will help you decide.

Most drugstores have shades that can work on a range of skin tones, so you can feel safe going a little lighter or darker. If you're stuck on whether to go lighter or darker, go lighter if you don't wear powder. Go darker if you like to wear powder. Setting powder over your foundation will make it look a bit lighter.

Hold the bottle to your jawline to get the closest match.

Try to go to the nearest and biggest window in the store. If you can't, then put your face and the bottle in front of a mirror.

Don't bother to put the bottle on your hand or wrist. It's always a bit darker.

Check the Guys' Aisle First

Men's products usually cost less, so you'll save on things such as deodorant, shaving cream, disposable razors, etc. Just stick with the unscented versions and your budget-saving secret is safe.

FREEBIE
For What It's Worth
Use the drugstore to get the latest color nail polish or other latest trend. Don't pay too much for anything you're not absolutely sure about.

HAIR PRODUCTS LIKE SHAMPOOS AND CONDITIONERS FROM DRUGSTORES ARE FINE. SOME ARE HIGHLY CONCENTRATED AND ARE BEST USED ON DAMP HAIR.

GENERIC BRANDS

Don't be married to name brands when it comes to certain products. Check the labeling. The best thing about many generic drug store items is their flexibility—buy one basic product and use it for several beauty treatments.

Petroleum Jelly

You can use it to moisturize your lips.

It's a great highlighter on top of cheekbones.

Add it to any powder eye shadow to create an eye gloss.

Spread it on cracked heels, elbows, and rough knees.

Baby Wipes

They are great makeup removers.

They clean stains.

Use them to refresh skin.

Cotton Swabs

They can be used to fix makeup mistakes.

Use them as emergency makeup applicators.

They are great tools for mixing colors.

GROCERY STORE BEAUTY FINDS

You can find great stuff in the kitchen or at the grocery store. For mere pennies, you can replicate very expensive cosmetics and skin care.

SKIP THE FANCY PACKAGING.

Use powdered milk in your bath to soften your skin.

Add brown sugar to your favorite shower gel to create your own body scrub.

PARSLEY

Get the dried variety or the fresh stuff. Put a teaspoon of the dried flakes in a cube and freeze it. Use it to get rid of the swelling in a pimple. Take a sprig of fresh parsley and chew it on your way out the door. Parsley is packed with chlorophyll, which is a major ingredient in breath mints.

LEMONS

Use the juice of a lemon mixed with an equal amount of water. It's a great oil-reducing facial toner.

Cut one up and put it in your bath for super clean skin and absolutely natural aromatherapy.

VEGETABLE BRUSH

Don't spend a lot on body brushes. A vegetable brush buffs away dead skin and gives a great glow at an affordable price. Use it on dry skin and just before showering.

BAKING SODA

Add enough water to baking soda to make a paste, and use it at night on blemishes to dry them up while you sleep.

Add it to your toothpaste to get rid of tartar and to whiten teeth.

KOSHER/SEA SALTS

Add your favorite essential oil to one-half cup of this coarse salt to make inexpensive bathing salts. Almond oil is a great choice. Or you might choose vanilla. You can even add a little food coloring. These make great gifts.

Use it on your scalp to get rid of dandruff. Before shampooing, massage damp scalp with about a tablespoon of salt.

DISCOUNT STORE DEALS

Burlington Coat Factory

Great leather buys, and, of course, lots of coats.

JC Penney

Very inexpensive casual wear. This store keeps up with trends and has regular sales on their top-selling items.

Kmart

They carry great workout wear. Check out the sports bras, shorts, and yoga pants. They come in a wonderfully soft cotton spandex and great colors!

189

Kohl's

They have a great juniors department with trendy stuff. Go up a size if you wear misses. Name brands can be found on sale regularly in the misses department.

Sears

They have a great private shoe line and quality basics like T-shirts, jeans, etc.

Target

Basics here can't be beat. The quality is high enough to really look great with the right accessorizing. Check out Mossimo and Stephen Sprouse if you're looking for trendier items.

Wal-Mart

I have personally switched over to their Faded Glory jeans. They're just as good as any of the designer brands I used to be loyal to. I love their basic T-shirts with just a bit of spandex. They carry the most extensive line of Hanes.

GREAT HAIR FOR LESS

HAIR CUTS

Here's a great way to get a great cut and spend little or nothing. Call around to large salons and ask if they have an apprentice or training night. If they do, that means you'll get a huge discount on cut, color, and blow dry. Don't be afraid. Every trainee is totally supervised.

HIGHLIGHTS

So you say you want to put highlights in your locks, but the expense is blocking your way? Do it gently with vinegar! Flavored vinegars can enhance and even create subtle highlights. You just choose the vinegar to match your hair.

Pale blonde…white vinegar

Deep blonde…balsamic vinegar

Strawberry blonde…raspberry vinegar

Dark Hair…red wine vinegar

Just add five tablespoons of vinegar to your shampoo. Leave it on for ten minutes. Then rinse. Condition if you need to. This solution is also great for shine and squeaky-clean hair.

USE A LITTLE SHAMPOO IN YOUR BATH FOR A TUB FULL OF BUBBLES.

BANG FOR YOUR BUCK

Mix your regular foundation with a pale, shimmery eye shadow like gold or beige. This is a good substitute for a very expensive shimmery foundation.

Always check the return policy of anything you're not absolutely sure about. Some stores offer full refunds even on opened or used products.

Look at ethnic skin lines if you need more pigment from your products since they tend to be more intense.

Dab a little antacid like Maalox on a pimple or cold sore.

FREE SAMPLES JUST FOR THE ASKING

Most cosmetic counters provide generous samples of skin care products, fragrances, and great little travel items like small tubes of lipstick. It's not something that is advertised, and counter people don't offer unless you ask.

Rather than just ask at each counter for anything free, pick a category. Ask about a fragrance you've seen. Look through the latest magazines. It's usually the newest products that have samples for customers to try.

Try not to go when it's very busy. That's when you'll have more one-on-one attention.

Don't ask, "What do you have for free?" and don't be greedy.

If you're really interested, you'll find you'll probably get better service and, after all, you might really like the products they're selling.

Chapter 18

CHEAP CHIC

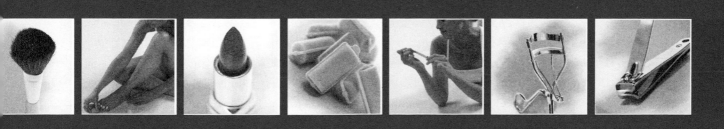

BARGAIN STYLE RULES

Don't think about what you wear too much. Polish your look with basic pieces, and then just go.

Just a little color goes a very long way. Don't overdo.

Never repeat outfits exactly. Do just one thing differently, and you'll greatly expand your wardrobe, as well as decrease your boredom factor.

A HEEL DRESSES UP ANY OUTFIT.

Anything black looks like it costs more.

Don't spend too much on anything overly trendy.

Shop in different departments than you usually shop (juniors, boys, men's, etc.)

Flea markets and thrift stores are chock-full of bargains.

A good pair of heels works with everything and makes it look like you paid more.

T-shirts are basics that know no class lines.

DON'T PUT DOWN A GREAT BUY BECAUSE IT'S MISSING A BUTTON OR HAS A PEN MARK. SHOW IT TO THE STORE MANAGER AND ASK FOR AN EXTRA DISCOUNT. JUST BE SURE TO FIX THE PROBLEM BEFORE YOU WEAR IT!

IT'S NO BARGAIN IF...

- It itches, chafes, or causes discomfort.
- It looks like it's been tried on just a few too many times.
- The color isn't right for you.
- You have nothing else to wear with it.

DISCOUNT STORE HINTS

Choose basic colors. Stores like Target always stock classic colors at incredibly inexpensive prices.

Know when a store gets in new merchandise. Ask the store manager when their truck makes deliveries.

STYLE BASICS

Work with what you've got (I'm talking about your body). The biggest bargain in any clothing is that you can use it to make figure flaws disappear. It's not what you wear; it's always how you wear it.

Big hips? Look for low-waisted pants. Coming right under the belly button, this cut will visually shrink hips. It also will make your torso look longer, and slims even further.

Hide thighs under a basic shirt-dress. It will glide right over those flaws. Just be sure to pick a fabric that's not too stiff (creating bulkiness), or too clingy.

Minimize a large bust by keeping brighter colors below the waist. Then the eye will naturally fall there.

Look slimmer all over by keeping with solid colors, including belts, scarf, etc.

NOBODY'S PERFECT AND YOU CERTAINLY DON'T HAVE TO ADVERTISE YOUR LESS-THAN-PERFECT BODY PARTS.

**Create an optical illusion with lines.
Vertical lines add height.
Horizontal lines add width.**

GET THE LOOK YOU WANT

SWEATERS

Trim your waist with a snug belted or wrap-around cardigan that defines the waist. Avoid oversized sweaters.

Get a flat tummy with a full-length sweater worn over a matching shell. Avoid body-hugging lightweight fabrics.

Trim hips with a brightly colored sweater that ends just above the hip. Avoid sweaters that fall just at or below the hip.

FREEBIE

Instant Chic

Pull a look together in seconds with a cardigan. It adds instant polish to slacks, skirts, and jeans. Duster length is the most flattering and versatile.

BRING ATTENTION TO THE UPPER HALF OF YOUR BODY WITH INTERESTING NECKLINES THAT DRAW THE EYE THERE.

BUY A CHEAP DENIM SKIRT AND CUT THE BOTTOM AT AN ANGLE OR STRAIGHT ACROSS AT THE HEM. THEN WASH AND DRY IT SO IT FRAYS. YOU'VE GOT INSTANT VINTAGE DENIM APPEAL.

PANTS

For a flatter tummy, look for flat-front pants that have a bit of Lycra. Avoid pockets and pleats.

For slimmer hips go for wide-leg pants in lightweight fabrics. Avoid prints or side pockets.

For longer legs choose pin stripes or slightly flared styles. Avoid cuffs or full legs.

For a smaller waist look for boot cut and a lowered waistband. Avoid baggy styles or high waists that end above the natural waistline.

Jeans Camouflage

Pick slightly relaxed dark denim jeans. If there are pockets on the jean, they should be close set. Don't wear your jeans too tight, or with too much stretch to them.

Choose pieces in sturdy fabrics like jersey, polyester, or dressy denim. They resist wrinkles so you can skip ironing.

Wrinkle-resistant fabric softeners, like Downy Enhancer, keep even more delicate fabrics looking freshly pressed.

PLUS-SIZED TRICKS

Don't wear tents and oversized clothing

Flaunt your curves by letting things skim, not stick.

Use three-quarter length items to add length and streamline.

Wear the proper undergarments. They should smooth out lines and support you.

Stay away from straight lines.

Bare what you like. The eye always goes first to the greatest exposure of skin.

OTHER SLIMMING TRICKS

One color head to toe.

Heels rather than flats.

Hose and shoes that match.

Belt and pants that match.

STAY AWAY FROM

Details where you don't want other eyes to stick.
Anything too tight just makes you look larger.
Large prints or plaids below the waist.
Pleats that don't lie flat.

USE COLOR

Just don't use so much that the first thing you see in the mirror is that color. It should be your face. You're safest saving the brightest colors as accents.

WHEN YOU FIND SOMETHING YOU LOVE AT A LOW PRICE, SNATCH IT UP IN EVERY COLOR AVAILABLE.

WHEN GOOD COLOR GOES WRONG

Large areas of light colors make figure flaws look bigger. Even black can be unflattering when it's shiny.

Think of a COLOR that makes you HAPPY. That's the one to go for. Wearing DIFFERENT SHADES of the same color GIVES YOU HEIGHT.

YOU CAN'T GO WRONG WITH NEUTRAL

A wardrobe built on neutrals, black, beige, navy, and brown mixes and matches in seconds. This makes it easy to grab and go and always look pulled together.

SHORTS FOR YOUR SHAPE

Disguise a tummy with flat-front shorts. Large thighs can look slimmer with shorts that cover the thigh and end above the knee. If you have short legs, wear shorts with vertical stripes.

SHOWING LESS TOP

If you want people to notice you, not your chest, rely on these tricks:

Choose dark-colored solid tops with high necklines. Dark colors take the emphasis away from the area.

Stay away from revealing necklines.

Stay away from anything that doesn't require a bra.

Skip stretchy fabrics.

Keep jewelry at the neckline or above.

INSTANT UPDATES FOR WHAT YOU ALREADY OWN

Breathe new life into what you already have in your closet before adding on.

SWEATERS

Dress up a basic cardigan by adding dressy button covers or sparkling rhinestones.

Add style to a long cardigan with a slim leather belt.

Take an ordinary crew neck sweater into a special event by pinning on a silk flower.

Bring sophistication to a V-neck sweater by adding a scarf at the neckline. Be sure to tuck the ends of the scarf into the neckline.

T-SHIRTS

Cut off the arms and show off your shoulders and a great tan.

Dress down a suit and dress up jeans with a basic black tee.

A narrow scoop neck tee provides an elegant neckline and backdrop for accessories.

A high-neck tee plays down a fuller bust.

A boatneck tee minimizes hips.

Relax V-necked tees bring the emphasis to the neck and away from the tummy.

FREEBIE

Dress up an inexpensive tee or skirt by sewing ribbon along the side seams. Or, attach an appliqué (Wal-Mart has a bunch to choose from). Most take just minutes to iron on.

NEVER CHIC (NO MATTER WHO SAYS SO)

Big baggy anything. Tents don't fool anyone. Slim is chic.

Too much jewelry.

Long dresses. You'll never get your money's worth.

SHOULD YOU KEEP IT, CAN YOU REINVENT IT?

KEEP IT

If you feel great every time you wear it. If it makes you happy just to look at it, even if it's not something that you wear very often, it's worth keeping.

If it has sentimental value. Sometimes a piece of clothing can bring memories back quicker than a snapshot. Keep these things in boxes, not in your closet.

If it's nothing to look at, but it's got a purpose. Certain pieces may not be glamorous, but you need those gloves, scarf, and rain boots.

TOSS IT

If it was expensive but you never wear it. It's just a reminder of money wasted. It serves no purpose except to make you feel bad.

If it doesn't fit. If something's too big or too small, it will just make you look bad when you wear it. It's not worth the closet space.

If you have several of the same. Do you really need ten black skirts? Take the top three and get rid of the rest. Sort them accordingly.

If it's the wrong color. If the color doesn't flatter you or it doesn't go with one other thing in your wardrobe, dump it. We all own those great buys in that awful "of course it's on sale because no one else would ever dream of wearing that" color.

If it hurts! There's nothing worse than something that's uncomfortable when you're wearing it. If your skin can't breathe, if it scratches or chafes, you need to throw it out.

If it's seen its better days. It may be classic, you may love it and have spent a fortune on it, but everything has a life. There's just so many times you can get something dry-cleaned, tailored, or resoled without it looking battered and spent.

FREEBIE

If you have a hard time getting rid of a piece of clothing, then move it to another part of the house. You should have a box for such items. Then, after a while, you'll be able to look through the box without being emotionally attached. You'll be ready to permanently get rid of the item.

BUYING RECYCLED

Shopping in thrift and vintage shops for recycled clothing can save you a bundle, but you need to know how to shop.

Check sizes. Vintage clothing tends to run smaller.

Look for flaws. Check zippers, seams, and hems. Hold the garment up to the light for holes and stains.

Don't bother with swimsuits and lingerie. They don't take use very well.

Pass up items that are unevenly faded.

SELLING RECYCLED

There are several Internet sites that you can use, like eBay and secondhand.com. There are also lots of ways you can make money on your castoffs in your own area.

Give it to a consignment shop.

Let someone else sell for you. Look in the Yellow Pages or on the web for this.

Rent a booth at a flea market. As the economy goes down, flea markets flourish. Since you'll probably do it only once, make sure everything is presentable. Group outfits together for an easier sale.

RECYCLING OLD JEWELRY

Take old clip-on earrings and dress up any pair of shoes or sandals.

A brooch looks great on an inexpensive handbag.

An old charm bracelet makes a purse look like a designer bag. Attach it handle to handle.

SEA SHELLS COLLECTED AT YOUR LAST VACATION MAKE GREAT JEWELRY FINDS AND ARE A STATEMENT OF YOUR INDIVIDUALITY. STRING SHELLS ON MICRO-CORDS OR CHAINS.

Chapter 19

ACCESSORIZING FOR LESS

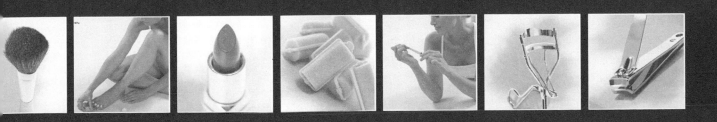

THE FINAL TOUCH

Accessorizing is the easiest, most inexpensive way to make a style statement.

THE PERFECT HANDBAG

It's such an important accessory, and so often overlooked. It's more visible than your shoes because it's closer to eye level for everybody to notice.

You don't need a bag that's more than 10 x 13 inches unless it's for business or travel.

It's not that important or necessary to match every outfit with an exactly matched bag. Actually, it makes you look like you're trying too hard. Pick a neutral color or a multi-colored bag if you want it to look like it goes with what you're wearing.

Find a handbag with one or two extra compartments to help you find things.

MATCHING **BAG** TO **BODY**

A small bag with a short shoulder strap will slim your hips and butt.

If you want to look less top heavy, let your bag fall at your waist or just below.

Look taller by locating a bag with a contrasting vertical detail.

Choose a bag that falls at the area that you consider your biggest asset, because that's where you'll be noticed.

LIGHTEN UP

It's not necessary to carry everything in your purse, and it's not practical to carry full-sized products. Don't ever have a bag so big that people ask you what you could possibly have in there.

BASIC NEEDS

Wallet

Keys

Breath mints

Comb/brush

Nail file

Tissues

Notebook & pen

A cosmetic bag with these essentials: lipstick (doubles as blush); foundation/powder combo; multi-use pencil for eyes, lips, brows.

DON'T TRY TO CARRY LOOSE POWDER in your purse

unless it's in a separate container. It just makes a mess.

WISE WALLETS

Consider a wallet's material first. Nylon is durable, easy to keep clean, and inexpensive.

Leather gets better as it ages. Calfskin is the best leather for wallets.

Light colors stain in any material don't wear well.

A leather change area is strongest.

Edges should be finished, not frayed.

Check for loose threads.

Test to make sure the metal tops of the wallet "kiss."

Test a zipper by tugging on the outside edges. Make sure it's strong and stays on track.

STORE YOUR COSMETICS

in a clear pencil case. In this way, you can see everything at a glance without having to dig. Keep a mirror in it, facing outward. Not only will you protect the mirror from getting dirty, but you'll also be able to see yourself at a glance.

SHOES

Not only are they an important accessory, they can create an entire look. Let's face it, the shoes stage the outfit.

GO FOR COMFORT

If you can't wear a pair of shoes comfortably for more than an hour, don't bother. Your face will show your pain, no matter how much makeup you apply.

There should be enough width to wiggle your toes.

The end of your longest toe should be about one-quarter to one-half inch from the end when you're standing.

The widest part of the shoe should fit the widest part of your foot comfortably.

The shoe should not slip when you walk.

Buy late in the day when your feet are largest.

Never buy a shoe that wrinkles when you flex your foot.

WEAR WHAT YOU LOVE
The shoes will dictate what follows.

FLATS LOOK BEST
with long skirts and slim pants.

SANDAL SOLUTIONS

The simpler the sandal, the more use you'll get.

Be sure the straps are well made, not too tight or too delicate.

Avoid sandals that cut any area of the foot.

Look for built-in arch support. Inner padding is the sign of a well-made sandal.

INEXPENSIVE SHOES
look richer in natural browns than in black.

BOOT BOOSTERS

Chunky boots need heavier hose. Don't wear sheer hose with boots.

Buy your size. Boots should be snug without cramping. Don't buy boots that are too big.

Don't stuff your calves into the boot. Look

for stretch materials if you have large calves.

Get non-skid soles from your shoemaker if your boots don't already have them.

HAT ADVICE

Never spend a lot for a hat. They blow away in the summer and take a beating in the rain and snow.

They're a great accessory, but not for everyone.

They look best outdoors.

Once you have a hat on, you need to keep it on. **HAT HEAD** is always a sure thing.

EYEGLASSES

Here's a great way to show off your style. Your glasses can make a major statement.

A long **narrow face** looks best in oval frames.

Cat's eye frames add width at the cheekbones.

Heart-shaped faces look best in oval or square frames, which hide width and create balance.

A **round face** is most flattered by an angled or squared shape since they add contours.

Soften a **square face** with round or oval frames. They help de-emphasize a strong jawline.

Shorten a **long nose** with light wire frames.

Aviator styles help slim a **broad face**.

HAIR CONSIDERATIONS

Gold rims bring out golden highlights.

Red or wine frames look great on redheads.

EYES

Tortoise shell is a good choice for brown eyes.

Blue eyes sparkle in clear or silver frames.

JEWELRY

The quickest way you can change your look is with jewelry. It's like a punctuation mark at the end of a sentence. The very same dress can become dressy with crystal jewelry, or go casual with wooden accessories.

EARRINGS

You can actually change the shape of your face with the right pair of earrings.

Larger earrings make the nose look smaller.

Avoid drop or shoulder earrings if you have a long face or short neck.

Colored stones can brighten your complexion.

Petites need delicate earrings.

Dangling earrings look best with short hair or up-dos.

Smaller earrings look best with glasses.

BELTS

The right belt can make you appear slimmer and taller. It can dress an outfit up or down.

A skinny belt can make your legs look longer. It draws the eye up; making your lower half look longer.

A thick middle can look smaller with a wide belt worn just below the waist. Wear it loosely.

Add height with a chain belt. Always wear it slung on your hips

WEAR ONLY ENOUGH JEWELRY TO **COMPLEMENT** YOUR OUTFIT, NOT **OVERWHELM** IT.

IF YOU WEAR A WIDE

BELT, let it rest on your hips. Wearing it

right at the waist will make the belt look

like a corset.

SUNGLASSES

A great accessory, but you've got to look at more than the style.

Plastic frames are less likely to pop out but scratch easily.

Polarized lenses filter out glare.

Mirrored lenses reflect it back.

Green works well in low and bright light.

Brown and amber are good for high glare or haze.

Gray, rose, and yellow are good for outdoor sports.

SCARVES

The perfect scarf can add glamour and polish to an otherwise dull look. There are many ways to use scarves.

Wear a scarf as a belt.

Use a scarf as a men's tie with a feminine touch.

Cheap scarves are a bargain buy. They double as belts and head wraps.

Chapter 20

DRESSING UP FOR LESS

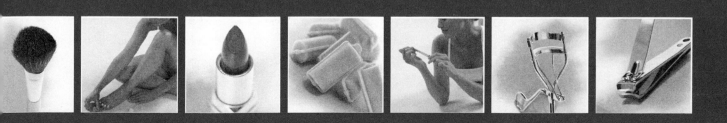

YOU DON'T HAVE TO SPEND A FORTUNE

You can still look like a million bucks with just a few changes. You don't want to spend a lot on special occasion clothing because you won't get enough use out of these specialty items. With a few adjustments you're on your way.

You can easily use your day wear when you:

- Dress up casual pants with dressy heels.
- Exchange your regular hose to fishnets or sheer and glittery hose.
- Change your leather belt to rhinestone, glitter, gold, or anything sparkly. Wear it with a sheath dress at hip-length.
- Use a rhinestone chain belt and dressy heels to dress up a pair of jeans.

DRESS UP THAT LITTLE BLACK SKIRT

If you own a basic black skirt (and who doesn't?), then there's never a need to stress over what to wear to that special event.

Add a matching V-neck top for simple sophistication.

Match hose and shoes.

DRESSING UP ON THE RUN

So many of us have to go from the office to that last-minute event. What's a girl to do? Not only do we not want to spend a lot, we don't have the time to spend it. Here's how you'll be prepared to head anywhere at anytime.

Always carry a pair of big sparkling earrings in your bag. If you have room, add a pendant.

Apply your makeup in the morning and simply intensify it just before heading out.

Carry a small tote with evening essentials, and keep the bag in good shape so that it can double as an evening bag to take with you.

Wash and blow dry your hair in the morning. Avoid using any styling products until you're ready to head out.

Keep a dressy pair of shoes in your car, perfectly polished.

If you don't have time to do your hair, just add a few rhinestone barrettes, or embellished bobby pins.

AN OLD BROOCH CAN MASK A STAIN.

A SILK FLOWER IS A GREAT way to dress up your hairdo. Use it in a ponytail or to pull back an unruly section of hair.

MAKING UP

LIGHTEN UP

Matte is for day. Your makeup should be as bright as the lights you'll be under.

Dip a wet brush in a bright eye shadow and use it to line eyes. This gives an intensity to the color, and it dries for longer wear.

KEEP YOUR MAKEUP GOING

Keep lips on all night by applying shimmery eye shadow on top of your lipstick. Apply in the middle of your upper and lower lips and spread out. Brighten your shadow by brushing on a layer of sheer white shadow first. Finish eyes and lips before adding blush so you can see how much you need to balance your look.

HAIR OCCASIONS

Curls are always in style for special events.

So are up dos, just make sure they don't have you looking like you're trying too hard. Twist your hair up loosely and pin it in place, leaving ends loose and pieces out around your face.

SEXY LOOKS FOR LESS

Look for inexpensive tube tops at malls as a good way of showing more skin. If you're really daring (as well as in good shape), you can even wear one as a skirt and create an amazing outfit.

Unbutton that extra button or two of any blouse.

Sheer tops that you usually wear a camisole with can be dressed up with a matching bra underneath.

SPECIAL FEATURES

ADD SOME SPARKLE

You can get away with dressing up just about anything you own with a little glitter. For example, a gold halter top dresses up a suit.

Stick to one embellished piece.

Wear it with something simple. For instance, wear a sequin top with black pants.

You don't need much jewelry when wearing anything sequined. One or two pieces are more than enough sparkle.

LACE IS LOVELY

Here's a fabric that can even take jeans into evening. Before making your purchase, check the flexibility of the lace. It should be soft and pliable to the touch. Discount stores have great sheer lace.

Any blouse can be dressed up with a lace collar and lace cuffs. Find them at fabric stores.

HOW TO WEAR SPAGHETTI STRAPS

Love wearing those little straps and sleeveless numbers, but no way are you going

to put out the big bucks for a special bra? Some fashionistas just let it all hang

out and match their bra straps with their tops. If this is not your style, then

wear your slimmest straps so that it looks like your top has more than one strap.

THE EVENING BAG

Everyday bags just can't make it into that special event. But you don't need to spend a lot of money on a bag that carries just a few essentials.

- Check the children's department. They have adorable versions of the most popular styles, perfectly sized for evening events.
- Use a cosmetic bag as an inexpensive, chic clutch.
- Take along one of those cute little bags that jewelry comes in.
- Dress up a pencil case with an elegant pin.
- You can even make your own evening bag with a remnant fabric or even a piece of an old prom gown or bridesmaid's gown. You just sew three sides together and add a cord as a drawstring.

- Don't forget to scour flea markets for vintage evening bags.

Chapter 21

FAST FIXES

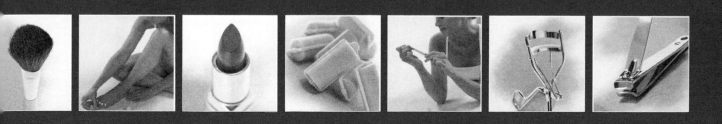

Beauty emergencies need to be solved as quickly as possible to get you out the door in a presentable style. Here are the most common emergencies with the quickest, most inexpensive way to treat them.

ACNE

This is the number one beauty emergency no matter how old you are. Deal with them on the "spot."

If the bump seems really red or swollen, apply an ice cube to reduce signs of inflammation.

To reduce redness, use an eye redness reliever or hydrocortisone. Hemorrhoid cream also works, all reduce the redness.

Dab on calamine lotion. It dries up and absorbs excess oil.

Mix one tablespoon of lemon juice and one tablespoon of cornstarch. Pat the paste on the blemish and let dry.

SHAVING NICKS

Moisten a dry tea bag with cold water and place it on the cut to stop the bleeding.

INSECT BITES

Mix one part meat tenderizer to four parts water and apply to bite.

SUNBURN

Chill a spray bottle of vinegar in the fridge, and then spray it on your burn.

Rub a peeled cucumber on the sunburn.

Pop an anti-inflammatory like ibuprofen.

Rub aloe vera gel on the burn.

POWDER OVERLOAD

Spritz your face with water and blot with a tissue for more natural coverage.

Take a clean, large fluffy brush and go over your face in circles.

QUICK GLOW FOR SALLOW SKIN

3 Minutes: Splash your face with as much cold water as you can handle about ten times. This gets blood flowing and invigorates skin.

2 minutes: Tap all over your face (lightly slapping yourself) until you feel your face tingle.

1 minute: Apply bronzing or shimmer powder on your forehead, cheeks, and chin.

30 seconds: Drop your head to the floor. This revs up circulation and puts color in your cheeks.

RED NOSE

Apply allergy drops with a cotton swab. Spread a mixture of green eye shadow and concealer to color-correct.

EYES

PUFFY EYES

Run teaspoons under cold water, and place them under your eyes for a few seconds. Then close your eyes and gently roll and massage the rounded side of the spoon over the eye area.

DARK CIRCLES

Apply sliced potatoes under the eye and lie down for five minutes, allowing the juices to seep in. Treat with the contents of a vitamin K capsule.

Mix bright blue shadow with facial moisturizer and dab it under your eyes with your finger.

TIRED/DROOPY EYES

A shimmer powder can visually lift droopy eyes. Use a cotton swab and apply it to the corner of the eyes.

HEAVY EYELINER

Go over the line with a light colored eye shadow to soften the look.

SMASHED EYE SHADOW

Store it in a small clean plastic or glass container and use it as a loose shadow.

LIPS

CHAPPED/DRY LIPS

Press tape against chapped lips and peel off dead skin cells.

MUSTACHE MENDING

If you waxed your upper lip and now it's pink and swollen, dip a washcloth in cold milk and press it to the area. This will soothe the skin, and lessen the inflammation.

SMEARED LIPSTICK

Dip a cotton swab in eye makeup remover. Apply foundation with a cotton swab to clean up the look.

NO TIME FOR MAKE UP

Apply a little bronzer to eyes, lips, and cheeks.

Use mascara in place of liner and shadow. A curling mascara will eliminate another step.

Stick to gloss and sheer lipsticks. They can be applied quickly without smudging.

HAIR EMERGENCIES

GREASIES

Blot your scalp with a baby wipe, followed by a tissue that's been pulled apart.

FRIZZIES

Mix equal amounts of conditioner and gel in your palms and run it over your hair. The gel will hold your style while the conditioner will control the frizz.

Pat moisturizer lightly over the top layer of hair.

NO TIME TO TOUCH UP ROOTS

Use colored sidewalk chalk.

Pat on powdered eye shadow.

NO TIME TO SHAMPOO

Pull hair into a low ponytail, leaving a few strands loose in front. Wash the strands and allow to dry. The strands will fake clean hair.

Shake a little cornstarch on your roots and brush through.

HAIR BUILD-UP

Get rid of fair build-up and bring hair back to life by adding a tablespoon of baking soda to two tablespoons of shampoo.

SPEEDY STYLES

QUICK DREADS

Divide your hair into one-inch sections and coat each with styling wax. Twist tightly around your finger. Repeat until your entire head is complete.

COILS

Wet hair and saturate with gel. Separate hair into one-inch sections and wrap tightly around a straw. Secure at the root to keep straws in place. Allow hair to dry or blow dry on the lowest setting. Slip out straws.

QUICK SHINE

After shampooing and conditioning, gently stroke hair from roots to ends with an ice cube. The cold seals the hair shaft, so it reflects light better.

Run a small amount of baby oil through your hair.

BROKEN LIPSTICK

- Put broken lipstick back together by heating the broken piece with a match until soft.

- Then sit it back on the tube, waiting five minutes before rolling it down the tube.

- Put it in the freezer for ten minutes to weld it together.

NO TIME TO BLOW DRY

Blow-dry only the hair on top of your head, above the ears. It's what frames your face and what people see first.

BLOW DRYER BURN OUT

Apply a few drops of castor oil with a grooming cream once hair is dry.

QUICK BANG TRIM

You can trim your own bangs. Start with dry bangs. Use the top half inch of a pair of small scissors with the blades angled upward, not across. Snip small pieces from side to side at least fifteen to twenty times.

TOO MUCH HAIR COLOR

If your hair came out too dark, shampoo with a mild dishwashing liquid. It will lift away some of the color pigment.

Shampoo with a dandruff shampoo, lathering twice.

TOO MUCH HAIR PRODUCT

Blot a witch hazel–soaked cotton ball over excess product to break down the product. Continue styling.

FAKE AN UP DO

Use a ponytail holder that looks like braided hair. Pull hair back into a low ponytail and twist into a bun. Secure with an elastic band and cover with holder.

EMERGENCY HAIR MOUSSE

Use a small amount of shaving cream (not shaving gel) in a fix.

CHLORINE-COLORED HAIR

Rinse with apple cider vinegar, followed by club soda.

Add three aspirin to a your regular shampoo dosage.

BAD HAIRCUT

Slick back with gel. Experiment with barrettes and headbands.

NAIL EMERGENCIES

YELLOW NAILS

Soak your nails in one-fourth cup of bleach mixed with one-half cup of water.

NO TIME FOR A MANICURE

Pass up the polish and give nails a quick buff with a nail file. They'll have smoothness and shine, and you won't have to wait for them to dry.

APPLY CLEAR LIP BALM TO NAILS FOR A POLISHED LOOK.

NOT QUITE DRY

Coat wet nails with cuticle oil and cover your nails with plastic wrap.

POLISH SMUDGE

Moisten the pad of your finger with polish remover and tap lightly to smooth it out.

CHIPPED POLISH

Moisten your finger with polish remover and quickly swipe over the chipped area to smooth out the edges.

BROKEN NAIL

If the break isn't too low, carefully cut the nail, file it, and trim the other nails so they're of equal length.

For a big break (one that's into the nail bed), apply a couple of drops of nail glue to the surface of the nail. Let set and hold the break in place for about a minute. Reapply glue and cover the nail with a piece of tea bag or tissue. Let dry, and then buff excess off.

POLISH BUBBLES

Go over the bubbles with a topcoat.

EMERGENCY NAIL POLISH REMOVERS

Use insect repellent when you need to remove your nail polish and there's none to be found.

Apply topcoat and rub off with a tissue.

CLOTHING EMERGENCIES

QUICK LINT REMOVER

Use sticky labels. They work faster than a skinny strip of tape.

BUTTON POPS

Strip the paper off a storage bag tie and use the metal to thread through the buttonhole. Twist it at the back to stay put.

Grab some dental floss and pass it through the hole where the button fell off, and through the buttonhole. Tie the ends together.

IF YOU RUN OUT OF FABRIC SOFTENER, PUT A COUPLE DROPS OF HAIR CONDITIONER ON A WASHCLOTH AND TOSS IT IN WITH THE CLOTHES.

PERSONAL EMERGENCIES

STOP HUNGER QUICKLY

Using a circular motion, rub the area between your upper lip and nose with your index finger for ten seconds. This fools the brain into signaling the stomach that it's satisfied.

GET A FLAT TUMMY

Keep away from carbonated beverages, even fizzy water, which can introduce air into the stomach.

Don't chew gum or sip from a straw because you'll swallow air.

Keep gas away by staying away from beans, cauliflower, peppers, and onions.

Chapter 22

BARGAIN TRAVEL SECRETS

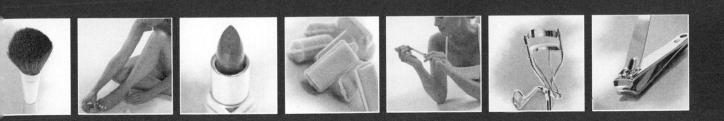

When you travel, you should look as polished and put together as you usually do. This takes a little extra time and effort, but can really make a big difference.

BE PREPARED

Keep your sample- and travel-sized items in a separate cosmetic bag ready to go. Resist the urge to use them at home.

Here are other "can't live without" items you need on the road:

Duct tape is a lifesaver when traveling. Take about a foot of it and wrap it around a pen or pencil. It will come in handy for lots of emergencies, such as:

Purse handle breaks

Sandal snaps

Emergency suitcase closure

Petroleum jelly stops skin chapping and chafing on planes, works to soothe sunburn, can tame flyaway hair, and can even polish shoes in an emergency.

Baby wipes can refresh makeup while on the road, remove stains, and refresh the skin when a shower is not an option.

LUGGAGE

Carry-on luggage, today more than ever, makes traveling so much easier. You only have to have experienced lost luggage once to want to keep your luggage with you. This is true even if you're going to be traveling for several days.

While the accepted maximum height for a carry-on is twenty-two inches, each airline has its own size restrictions. Checking ahead is always a good idea.

FEATURES TO LOOK FOR

Details to look for in selecting a rolling carry-on bag include a sturdy handle and ball-bearing or in-line skate wheels.

Look for fabrics that are lightweight yet sturdy, like nylon, canvas, or a sturdy polyester blend, and make sure the fabric has been coated to repel moisture.

An added benefit is to choose a bag with a strap that enables you to piggyback another smaller bag on top.

Try to get a manufacturer's warranty of at least three years.

Forget bags with multiple compartments. You'll fit more in an empty box-style carrier.

KEEP YOUR LUGGAGE SAFE

Since most of the luggage sold is black, it can easily be confused with someone else's, especially on the conveyer belt at the baggage claim. Try to choose a color that no one else has. And yes, the hot pink and green luggage colors are the ones usually on sale.

If you already own black luggage, identify it as yours with a colorful scarf or a bright ribbon.

Label your luggage inside and out. Be sure to include your destination address and phone number as well.

PACKING

Packing requires discipline and restraint. Always pack the least amount of clothing, shoes, and cosmetics that you think you need to survive.

LEARN TO DO MORE WITH LESS
You really only need a few well-planned pieces.

IN THE CARRY-ON

If you do have to check your luggage, assume it may not make the destination with you, and carry your absolute essentials with you at all times.

If you wear contact lenses, keep the necessary solutions and containers with you.

Always keep some extra underwear and hose in a plastic bag in your purse.

If you do check your luggage, consider having it shrink-wrapped. It keeps luggage from popping open and it deters thieves. You can easily do it yourself to save money. Just use wide plastic wrap and two-inch cellophane tape.

KNOW WHAT **NOT TO BRING**

Check out the weather of where you'll be traveling to on the Internet.

Call your hotel to make sure that they have hair dryers and irons so you don't have to pack them.

Also ask your hotel if they will provide a robe in your room. It also doubles as a beach cover-up.

CHOOSE DARK COLORS

They hide spots and wrinkles. Use two colors at the very most for easy mix and matching with fewer pieces.

BREAK IT UP

Pantsuits and skirt suits should be considered separates.

ACCESSORIES

Choose a purse that can fit inside your briefcase.

Never carry a purse so large that it looks like you're living out of it.

Pack accessories that can take an office look into evening like rhinestones and crystal jewelry.

Interlock belts and run them along your suitcase's inner circumference to save space.

SHOES

Wear mules (backless shoes) if you need to wear heels while traveling by air. They can easily be slipped off on the plane, and can still fit at the end of the trip when your feet have swollen considerably.

Always include walking shoes

A light pair of evening shoes with a comfortable heel is ideal, but if you have no room, bring a pair of clip-on earrings to dress up your day shoes.

Before packing a CD player or other battery-operated item, put the batteries in the wrong way. In this way, if the appliance is accidentally switched on, the batteries won't be drained.

PACK WELL

A black dress is a versatile go-anywhere-in-any-kind-of-climate staple. The simpler the styling, the more looks you'll be able to create with it. Choose one with just a hint of stretch to flatter without clinging.

Fold clothes where the natural creases would be, like elbows and knees.

Keep your clothing in its dry cleaning bags if there's room. The plastic forms air pockets that will keep clothing from being crushed.

Leave your bulkiest clothing out and wear it on the plane.

Place shoes and heavier items (like blue jeans) at the bottom of your bag when you pack.

Stuff your shoes with socks, medicine, film, and jewelry.

Roll your clothing whenever possible to avoid wrinkling.

Put your shoes in plastic bags to protect clothing.

Wrap your dressier clothing around something soft (like a beach towel).

Always unpack and hang your clothing immediately upon arrival.

BIGGER IS NOT ALWAYS BETTER when it comes to luggage. If you don't fill your suitcase, your clothing will fall all over the place, which will cause wrinkling and make a big, jumbled mess.

BASICS

Here is a list of seasonless wardrobe essentials that can be combined in many ways.

Tops
T-shirt
Tank top
Sweater or cardigan

231

WRINKLE-PROOFING

These fabrics will wrinkle less than others:

- NYLON AND NYLON-SPANDEX BLENDS

- POLYESTER

- VISCOSE

- MICRO FIBERS

- RAYON AND COTTON BLENDS

- SILK

- KNITS

Bottoms

A skirt: Pack one in a neutral color and basic style and length.

Pants: The most comfortable to wear on the plane is a pair of stretch pants. Your second pair should able to work as city day wear or at an evening dinner.

IF WEATHER PERMITS

Bring a swimsuit. It doesn't take much room and there may be an indoor pool, even if you're staying in the city.

If you feel comfortable in a bikini, the top can work with pants or shorts. Pack a big shirt to act as a cover up or jacket.

IF YOU WORK OUT

Shorts
Sports bra
Tank top
Sneakers/socks

BEAUTY ON THE ROAD

While traveling, you should try to maintain your beauty routine in the usual way with a few extra touches.

Drink at least eight ounces of water every hour. The dry air on planes (not to mention the lack of oxygen) is like being stranded in a desert.

If you can, wear a sleep mask while traveling. Some are scented with soothing herbs, while others are lightly weighted to reduce puffiness. Some masks have a cooling effect.

Travel with a satin pillowcase so you won't wake up with morning creasing.

HEALTH ON THE ROAD

Whether in a car or plane, use a pillow you can roll up for lumbar or neck support.

Do heel raises, ankle circles, toe lifts, and overhead stretches every hour in flight to avoid cramping. Take a walk up and down the aisle once an hour to work the leg muscles and ease the back!

Prevent air bloating by leaning forward in your seat and supporting your face in your hands for several minutes. You're providing the right amount of pressure on your facial tissue to combat puffiness.

Avoid high sodium snacks while in the air.

Tense each muscle in your body then release it and relax completely.

Breathe through your nose to defend against cabin germs.

Work out in the comfort and safety of your hotel room. Use wine bottles from the mini bar as free weights.

SAFETY ON THE ROAD

HOTELS

Choose hotels with interior room entrances and avoid hotels with hallways that lead to a parking lot or maintenance area.

Pick a hotel location where transportation and security is readily available.

A smaller hotel and lobby is safer than a large hotel since staff will notice strangers and loiterers more easily.

Always ask for a higher floor. Never accept a first-floor room.

Ask that your room number be written down, not spoken.

Book a room close to the elevator.

Use the Do Not Disturb sign even while you're out of your room.

Leave the TV or radio and lights on to give the impression that there is someone in the room.

Check your windows, sliding doors, and locks.

Use the door chain when you're in your room.

Close your curtains.

Bring along a rubber doorstop for extra security while you sleep. They're especially useful for providing security on doors in adjoining rooms.

Always check with the front desk before opening the door to anyone.

CAR TRAVEL

Wear driving slippers or comfortable shoes whether you're the driver or passenger.

Use sun block with an SPF of at least 30. Sun rays have the ability to penetrate glass.

Dress in layers for a car trip. It may be chilly in the morning but can get hot by late afternoon. Dressing in layers will eliminate the need to go searching through your luggage once you're on the road.

Bring along a small cooler with bottled water and healthy snacks. It will keep you from being tempted by the bright lights of the fast food restaurants you're driving past.

CELEBRITY TRAVEL SECRETS

Since celebrities practically live on the road, they have by default become experts at travel. The products they can't live without are inexpensive but absolutely essential to these stars.

Talk show host **Ananda Lewis** carries olive oil and uses it on her hair and body straight from the bottle.

Singer **Britney Spears** won't leave home without Herbal Essences volumizing shampoo.

Actress **Gretchen Mol** uses Elizabeth Arden Ceramide capsules to give her face a glow.

Janet Jackson pops Castile soap in her bag.

It's something her mom has always used and everyone in the family carries it when they travel.

Claire Danes likes the free products that she gets at the Four Seasons hotels, especially their shampoo.

Lisa Kudrow uses collagen patches on her eyes while flying.

Mariel Hemingway brings evening primrose oil with her when she travels. It not only strengthens and adds shine to her hair; she claims it gives her complexion more elasticity. It's available in capsules everywhere.

Alexandra Paul carries psyllium husk to prevent constipation while she's traveling and eating on the road.

Providence star **Melina Kanakaredes** keeps her lips moist and smooth with hoof cream when she's traveling. (Yes, it was originally formulated for horses' hooves!)

Shania Twain never travels without Bag Balm, made to keep cows' udders from getting sore while they're being milked. Her skin tends to dry out when she's flying, so she rubs it over her entire face to protect it.

Lucy Liu carries lavender oil to keep her calm and relaxed in-flight.

Fashion designer **Adrienne Vittadini**'s favorite travel item is a shawl. She uses it on planes, for cool evenings as a wrap, and in air-conditioned offices. She also shares that she won't allow hotels to iron her clothing because she finds them too heavy-handed. Instead, she wraps each item in tissue paper and then steams them in the shower in her hotel room.

Supermodel **Naomi Campbell** travels with two bottles of hot sauce, Jamaican and domestic to keep her metabolism fired up, and for low-calorie snacking while on the road.

Claudia Schiffer takes turkey jerky along with her as a high-protein, practically fat-free snack. It takes a while to eat and is easy to carry.

SECURITY TIME SAVERS

Don't wear any metal jewelry on the day of your flight. Try not to even wear an underwire bra. In an age of tightened security, assume that *anything* will set off a metal detector.

Before entering the airport, tuck your ID in a secure pocket that you can access quickly.

JET LAG PREVENTION

Don't drink caffeinated, carbonated, or alcoholic beverages if you plan to sleep.

If you travel east, get a half hour of sun when you awaken.

If you travel west, get your sun late in the day.

Bring earplugs to block out sounds. Moldable foam ones work best.

Check with your doctor about taking melatonin.

AIRLINE SERVICE TIPS

When booking your flight, avoid the front row or bulkhead. This is where infants are generally seated.

Don't stow your bag in an overhead bin behind you. Otherwise you'll have to fight the flow of traffic to get to your bag.

When flying on a weekday, fly early in the day. That's when most airlines post the fewest delays.

FINAL WORDS

It has been my intent in this book to allow beauty to become more attainable, understandable, and more affordable for everyone. The beauty and diet industries know how to push our buttons by playing to our emotions, causing us to look for that magic elixir. There is no one answer. Each technique, each trick, every product should help lead you to the eventual goal: better looks and more confidence.

If you find that some of the techniques take some time to master, don't worry. Once you've conquered the learning curve, you will be delighted by the remarkable results as much as the substantial savings. There are more options than ever in beauty and diet. Explore as many as your lifestyle will allow. Then, adopt what you enjoy and what works best.

I'm always here to help. Bringing out beauty in women of every age, size, ethnicity, and background is my privilege. Please write to me via my website at dianeirons.com and let me know your issues. As always, I am deeply honored that you have allowed me into your life.

SITES & RESOURCES

FREEBIES

They say cheap is good. Well how about free? Cosmetics counters give away samples to get their customers hooked. Here's a sampling of some of the companies that regularly offer samples at their counters.

If you are able to engage the counter person, and you catch her at a slow time, she may even take time to apply some of her newest products on you. Of course, they would like you to buy on the spot, but you're not under any obligation. The best way to gracefully get away is to simply and honestly tell her that you need to see everything out in the sunlight and see if the product suits you.

Calvin Klein
Chanel
Clarins
Clinique
Elizabeth Arden
Estée Lauder
Lalique
Nars
Orlane
Prada
Prescriptives
Sisley
Yves Saint Laurent

There's always more. Just ask if there's a sample, while looking over a product that interests you.

There's definitely an etiquette involved to getting free stuff. What you don't want to do is to go from counter to counter with a big Halloween type bag and a "trick or treat" kind of attitude.

Bring in an ad from a magazine. Chances are, if it's a new product that's being introduced, there's a sample.

SITE SAMPLES

Here are some sites I've come across that I thought you might enjoy.

SHOPPING ADVICE SITES

www.fashionmall.com
www.focusonstyle.com
www.TheTrendReport.com
www.Saleshound.com
www.salesmountain.com
www.inshop.com
www.Dailyshopper.com
www.internetmall.com

DESIGNER SITES

www.chanel.com
www.ArmaniExchange.com
www.donnakaran.com

SHOPPING SITES

www.GUESS.com
www.gap.com
www.bluefly.com
www.girlshop.com
www.bestpromdresses.com
www.turnstylz.com

www.styleshopdirect.com
www.net-a-porter.com
www.styleshop.com
www.zappos.com

FUN SITES

www.astrologyfashion.com
www.quackwatch.com

BEAUTY SITES

www.Beautycare.com
www.Emakemeup.com
www.Profaces.com
www.beautyofasite.com
www.beautyscene.com
www.ezface.com

SKIN ADVICE SITES

www.pimpleportal.com
www.dermadoctor.com

HAIR SITES

www.Robertcraig.com
www.Salonweb.com

FOOD & FITNESS SITES

www.ediets.com (This site has diet support as well as message boards where members support one another.)
www.whymilk.com
www.ideafit.com (This organization is for fitness pros and fitness enthusiasts.)
www.acefitness.com (Sends health and fitness news to anyone interested in finding late-breaking information.)
www.videofitness.com (Women share information about good/bad fitness videos.)

BODY/HEALTH INFORMATION

www.tampax.com
www.eatright.org. (Everything you need to maintain a healthy eating style. A daily tip is offered on the site's home page.)

PRODUCT REVIEW SITES

www.Epinions.com

SWIMSUIT HELP SITES

www.jantzenswim.com

GOOD CAUSES

www.shoesforafrica.com (This site gives new life to your worn-out running shoes. Shoes for Africa gives old athletic shoes to needy people in Africa.)

www.thewomensalliance.org (This organization accepts professional attire which should be cleaned before donating.)
www.bottomlesscloset.org (This organization accepts office-appropriate clothing.)

HELP HOTLINES

Suicide & Crisis Hotline (800) 999-9999
National Suicide Prevention (877) 727-4747
American Dietetic Association (800) 366-1655
American Anorexia/Bulimia Association Inc.
(212) 501-8351
239 Central Park West
Suite 1R
New York, NY 10024
National Association of Anorexia and Associated Disorders
(847) 831-3438
PO Box #7
Highland Park, IL 60035

INDEX

ABOUT THE AUTHOR

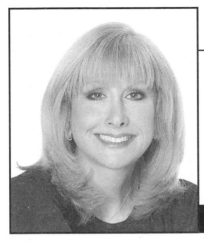

DIANE IRONS began her career as a model at age fourteen, then moved on to become a highly successful journalist and internationally known fashion and image expert. Her consumer approach to beauty, diet, and cosmetics has helped thousands of women realize that glamour and style are every woman's birthright and should be inexpensive and fun. She lives in the Boston area.

For more on Diane visit her website at dianeirons.com.